John T. Pardeck, PhD
Charles F. Longino, Jr., PhD
John W. Murphy, PhD
Editors

Reason and Rationality in Health and Human Services Delivery

Reason and Rationality in Health and Human Services Delivery has been co-published simultaneously as *Journal of Health & Social Policy*, Volume 9, Number 4 1998.

"**I**f those deeply steeped in the assumptions, canons and traditions of the Western biomedical model of medicine read this book, it is likely that some major changes in American health care will take place. Pardeck, Longino and Murphy have pulled together in seven chapters a variety of perspectives that successfully challenge the pillars of modern medicine including dualism, reason and the fashion in which medical decisions are made. Their analysis, and that of others, of dualism, reason and decision making as it takes place in a postmodern world lead to a completely different method of understanding medical reality and the treatment flowing therefrom. The overall implicit assertion of this book is that the practice of modern medicine and the education of its practitioners lags behind developments in other professions and disciplines. This is particularly true for the manner in which medicine conducts its scientific research. Of the major professions it is only in medicine that the belief in a value free science persists along with separation of the person from the disease. This book will provide intellectual ammunition for health care advocates throughout the United States who are working diligently to regulate the pervasiveness of managed care systems and the disempowerment of persons caught up in them. As the person/patient becomes empowered and a participant in the process of diagnosis and treatment, a new and more relevant process of reason and rationality in medical care will emerge. This book should be required [reading] of all health care professionals, especially those training to become physicians."

Roland Meinert, PhD
President
Missouri Association for Social Welfare

More pre-publication
REVIEWS, COMMENTARIES, EVALUATIONS . . .

"**T**his [volume] illuminates beautifully how helping professionals must consult the life-world of individuals in order to enhance health care in the United States. Posited within the context of postmodernism, the authors in this book make a strong case for the notion that reason and rationality in health and human service delivery is found in the perceptions of patients and/or consumers of services. One author suggests that only by empowering the patient can health care in this country be improved; another author suggests this can be accomplished when researchers work with community members to understand the context and meaning of a community and thus its members. Perhaps the most powerful chapters in the manuscript are those that demonstrate how the very real human experiences of patients, service providers, and organizations are contextual and, in some sense, context provides the basis for making health and human service delivery more rather than less rational.

. . . . [T]he authors give perspectives on health and human services delivery that bring into question the extent to which the delivery system is rational, especially within the context [of] managed care that all but excludes both service provider and consumer in the decision-making process. The fact that the authors question what is rational about the current system is exhilarating and courageous–to say nothing of informative. Each and every chapter takes the reader on a journey into a health and human service delivery system that could be if society accepts the perceptions of patients/clients as the basis for their reality and potential for empowerment."

Martha Markward, PhD
School of Social Work
University of Georgia

The Haworth Press, Inc.

Reason and Rationality in Health and Human Services Delivery

Reason and Rationality in Health and Human Services Delivery has been co-published simultaneously as *Journal of Health & Social Policy,* Volume 9, Number 4 1998.

The *Journal of Health & Social Policy* Monographs/"Separates"

Health Care for the Poor and Uninsured: Strategies that Work, edited by Nellie P. Tate and Kevin T. Kavanagh

Psychological Aspects of Sickle Cell Disease: Past, Present, and Future Directions of Research, edited by Kermit B. Nash

Selected Practical Problems in Health and Social Research, edited by Thomas E. Dinero

Reason and Rationality in Health and Human Services Delivery, edited by John T. Pardeck, Charles F. Longino, Jr., and John W. Murphy

These books were published simultaneously as special thematic issues of the *Journal of Health & Social Policy* and are available bound separately. Visit Haworth's website at http://www.haworth.com to search our online catalog for complete tables of contents and ordering information for these and other publications. Or call 1-800-HAWORTH (outside US/Canada: 607-722-5857), Fax: 1-800-895-0582 (outside US/Canada: 607-771-0012), or e-mail getinfo@haworth.com

Reason and Rationality in Health and Human Services Delivery

John T. Pardeck, PhD
Charles F. Longino, Jr., PhD
John W. Murphy, PhD
Editors

Reason and Rationality in Health and Human Services Delivery has been co-published simultaneously as *Journal of Health & Social Policy,* Volume 9, Number 4 1998.

The Haworth Press, Inc.
New York • London

Reason and Rationality in Health and Human Services Delivery
has been co-published simultaneously as *Journal of Health & Social Policy*, Volume 9, Number 4 1998.

The development, preparation, and publication of this work has been undertaken with great care. However, the publisher, employees, editors, and agents of The Haworth Press and all imprints of The Haworth Press, Inc., including The Haworth Medical Press and The Pharmaceutical Products Press, are not responsible for any errors contained herein or for consequences that may ensue from use of materials or information contained in this work. Opinions expressed by the author(s) are not necessarily those of The Haworth Press, Inc.

The Haworth Press, Inc., 10 Alice Street, Binghamton, NY 13904-1580 USA

Cover design by Thomas J. Mayshock Jr.

Library of Congress Cataloging-in-Publication Data

Reason and rationality in health and human services delivery / John T. Pardeck, Charles F. Longino, John W. Murphy, editors.
        p. cm.
"Co-published simultaneously as Journal of health & social policy, v. 9, no. 4, 1998."
Includes bibliographical references and index.
ISBN 0-7890-0509-3 (alk. paper)
        1. Medical care–Philosophy. 2. Medical ethics. I. Pardeck, John T. II. Longino, Charles R., 1938- . III. Murphy, John W. IV. Journal of health and social policy.
RA427.25.R43 1998
362.1'01–dc21   98-10498
                                                                                                              CIP

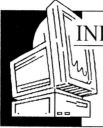

INDEXING & ABSTRACTING

Contributions to this publication are selectively indexed or abstracted in print, electronic, online, or CD-ROM version(s) of the reference tools and information services listed below. This list is current as of the copyright date of this publication. See the end of this section for additional notes.

- *Abstracts in Anthropology*, Baywood Publishing Company, 26 Austin Avenue, P.O. Box 337, Amityville, NY 11701

- *Academic Abstracts/CD-ROM,* EBSCO Publishing Editorial Department, P.O. Box 590, Ipswich, MA 01938-0590

- *BIOBUSINESS:* covers business literature related to the life sciences; covers both business & life science periodicals in such areas as pharmacology, health care, biotechnology, foods & beverages, etc., BIOSIS, Bibliographic Control Department, 2100 Arch Street, Philadelphia, PA 19103-1399

- *Cambridge Scientific Abstracts, Health and Safety Science Abstracts,* 7200 Wisconsin Avenue #601, Bethesda, MD 20814

- *CNPIEC Reference Guide: Chinese National Directory of Foreign Periodicals*, P.O. Box 88, Beijing, People's Republic of China

- *Excerpta Medica/Secondary Publishing Division*, Elsevier Science Inc., Secondary Publishing Division, 655 Avenue of the Americas, New York, NY 10010

- *Family Studies Database (online and CD/ROM),* National Information Services Corporation, 306 East Baltimore Pike, 2nd Floor, Media, PA 19063

- *GEO Abstracts (GEO Abstracts/GEOBASE)*, Elsevier/GEO Abstracts, Regency House, 34 Duke Street, Norwich NR3 3AP, England

- *Health Care Literature Information Network/HECLINET*, Technische Universitat Berlin/Dokumentation Krankenhauswesen, Sekr. A42, Strasse des 17. Juni 135, D 10623 Berlin, Germany

- *Health Management Information Service (HELMIS),* Nuffield Institute for Health, 71-75 Clarendon Road, Leeds LS2 9PL, England

- *Health Source: Indexing & Abstracting of 160 selected health related journals, updated monthly:* EBSCO Publishing, 83 Pine Street, Peabody, MA 01960

- *Health Source Plus: expanded version of "Health Source" to be released shortly:* EBSCO Publishing, 83 Pine Street, Peabody MA 01960

(continued)

- *Healthcare Marketing Abstracts*, COR Research, Inc., P.O. Box 40959, Santa Barbara, CA 93140-0959
- *HealthPromis*, Health Education Authority (HEA)/Health Promotion Information Centre, Hamilton House-Mabledon Place, London WC1H 9TX, England
- *HealthSTAR*, National Library of Medicine, 8600 Rockville Pike, Bethesda, MD 20894
- *Hospital and Health Administration Index*, American Hospital Association, One North Franklin, Chicago, IL 60606
- *IBZ International Bibliography of Periodical Literature*, Zeller Verlag GmbH & Co., P.O.B. 1949, d-49009, Osnabruck, Germany
- *Index to Periodical Articles Related to Law*, University of Texas, 727 East 26th Street, Austin, TX 78705
- *International Political Science Abstracts*, 27 Rue Saint-Guillaume, F-75337 Paris, Cedex 07, France
- *INTERNET ACCESS (& additional networks) Bulletin Board for Libraries ("BUBL"), coverage of information resources on INTERNET, JANET, and other networks.*
  - <URL:http://bubl.ac.uk/>
  - The new locations will be found under <URL:http://bubl.ac.uk/link/>.
  - Any existing BUBL users who have problems finding information on the new service should contact the BUBL help line by sending e-mail to <bubl@bubl.ac.uk>.
  The Andersonian Library, Curran Building, 101 St. James Road, Glasgow G4 0NS, Scotland
- *Medical Benefits*, P.O. Box 1007, Charlottesville, VA 22902
- *Medication Use STudies (MUST) DATABASE*, The University of Mississippi, School of Pharmacy, University, MS 38677
- *Mental Health Abstracts (online through DIALOG)*, IFI/Plenum Data Company, 3202 Kirkwood Highway., Wilmington, DE 19808
- *National Clearinghouse for Primary Care Information (NCPCI)*, 2070 Chain Bridge Road, Suite 450, Vienna, VA 22182-2536
- *NIAAA Alcohol and Alcohol Problems Science Database (ETOH)*, National Institute on Alcohol Abuse and Alcoholism, 1400 Eye Street NW, Suite 600, Washington, DC 20005
- *OT BibSys*, American Occupational Therapy Foundation, P.O. Box 31220, Rockville, MD 20824-1220
- *Public Affairs Information Bulletin (PAIS)*, Public Affairs Information Service, Inc., 521 West 43rd Street, New York, NY 10036-4396
- *Sage Public Administration Abstracts (SPAA)*, Sage Publications, Inc., 2455 Teller Road, Newbury Park, CA 91320
- *Social Planning/Policy & Development Abstracts (SOPODA)*, Sociological Abstracts, Inc., P.O. Box 22206, San Diego, CA 92192-0206

(continued)

- *Social Work Abstracts*, National Association of Social Workers, 750 First Street NW, 8th Floor, Washington, DC 20002
- *Sociological Abstracts (SA)*, Sociological Abstracts, Inc., P.O. Box 22206, San Diego, CA 92192-0206
- *UP-TO-DATE Publications*, 3160 Steeles Avenue East, Suite 215, Markham, Ontario L3R 4G9, Canada
- *World Agricultural Economics & Rural Sociology Abstracts, c/o CAB International/CAB ACCESS . . . available in print, diskettes updated weekly, and on INTERNET. Providing full bibliographic listings, author affiliation, augmented keyword searching,* CAB International, P.O. Box 100, Wallingford Oxon OX10 8DE, United Kingdom

SPECIAL BIBLIOGRAPHIC NOTES

*related to special journal issues (separates)
and indexing/abstracting*

☐ indexing/abstracting services in this list will also cover material in any "separate" that is co-published simultaneously with Haworth's special thematic journal issue or DocuSerial. Indexing/abstracting usually covers material at the article/chapter level.

☐ monographic co-editions are intended for either non-subscribers or libraries which intend to purchase a second copy for their circulating collections.

☐ monographic co-editions are reported to all jobbers/wholesalers/approval plans. The source journal is listed as the "series" to assist the prevention of duplicate purchasing in the same manner utilized for books-in-series.

☐ to facilitate user/access services all indexing/abstracting services are encouraged to utilize the co-indexing entry note indicated at the bottom of the first page of each article/chapter/contribution.

☐ this is intended to assist a library user of any reference tool (whether print, electronic, online, or CD-ROM) to locate the monographic version if the library has purchased this version but not a subscription to the source journal.

☐ individual articles/chapters in any Haworth publication are also available through the Haworth Document Delivery Service (HDDS).

Reason and Rationality in Health and Human Services Delivery

CONTENTS

ABOUT THE EDITORS

John T. Pardeck is Professor of Social Work in the School of Social Work at Southwest Missouri State University. He received his MSW and PhD in social work from St. Louis University. Pardeck has published over 100 articles in academic and professional journals. His most recent books include *Computers in Human Services: An Overview for Clinical and Welfare Services* (with John W. Murphy) (1990, Harwood Academic Publishers), *The Computerization of Human Services Agencies: A Critical Appraisal* (with John W. Murphy) (1991, Auburn House), *Issues in Social Work: A Critical Analysis* (with Roland G. Meinert and William P. Sullivan) (1994, Auburn House), and *Social Work Practice: An Ecological Approach* (1996, Auburn House).

Charles F. Longino, Jr., received his PhD from the University of North Carolina. Currently he is Professor of Sociology and Director of the Reynolda Gerontology Program at Wake Forest University. Dr. Longino's research interests include gerontology and medical sociology. He has published 117 articles, chapters, or encyclopedia entries, 14 books, monographs, and compendia. His most recent books include *Retirement Migration in America* and, with John W. Murphy, *The Old Age Challenge to the Biomedical Model.*

John W. Murphy received his PhD from Ohio State University. Currently he is Professor of Sociology at the University of Miami, Coral Gables, FL. Dr. Murphy's most recent books are *The Politics of Culture* and *Postmodernism, Unraveling Racism, and Democratic Institutions.*

Reason and Rationality in Health and Human Services Delivery: An Introduction

John T. Pardeck, PhD, ACSW
Charles F. Longino, Jr., PhD
John W. Murphy, PhD

The reader may ask, why devote a volume to what might appear to be esoteric topics, reason and rationality? A simple answer is that these topics, for some time, have been at the center of the Western intellectual tradition. Furthermore, appeals are made regularly to increased rationality to enhance the delivery of health care and social services. The claim is that service delivery will be improved appreciably if planning and implementation of services is made more rigorous.

Reason has been the centerpiece of most of Western philosophy. At one time or another, reason has been understood to either ground knowledge, substantiate morals, or guarantee the proper deployment of history. Truth, fact, and order, moreover, have all been linked to reason. And in more modern times, science and advanced technology, such as computers, have been identified as having privileged access to reason. For example, the use of computer technology in modern medicine is thought to epitomize ratio-

John T. Pardeck is Professor of Social Work, School of Social Work at Southwest Missouri State University, Springfield, MO 65804. Charles F. Longino, Jr., is Director of the Reynolda Gerontology Program and Professor of Sociology at Wake Forest University, Winston-Salem, NC 27109. John W. Murphy is Professor of Sociology at the University of Miami, Coral Gables, FL 33124.

[Haworth co-indexing entry note]: "Reason and Rationality in Health and Human Services Delivery: An Introduction." Pardeck, John T., Charles F. Longino, Jr., and John W. Murphy. Co-published simultaneously in *Journal of Health & Social Policy* (The Haworth Press, Inc.) Vol. 9, No. 4, 1998, pp. 1-8; and: *Reason and Rationality in Health and Human Services Delivery* (ed: John T. Pardeck, Charles F. Longino, Jr., and John W. Murphy) The Haworth Press, Inc., 1998, pp. 1-8. Single or multiple copies of this article are available for a fee from The Haworth Document Delivery Service [1-800-342-9678, 9:00 a.m. - 5:00 p.m. (EST). E-mail address: getinfo@haworth.com].

nality and guarantee the most efficient use of services which allows the human presence to be removed categorically from reason (Longino & Murphy, 1995). As a result, subjectivity, or any other variant of interpretation, is thought to influence negatively the exercise of rationality. In general, reason is seen as immune to the contaminants that plague other modes of knowledge and practice.

Reason is thus seen as positive by most everyone. Virtually every undertaking is thought to be upgraded by practices that enhance rationality. Research methodologies, laboratory techniques, or intervention strategies that reflect reason are presumed to facilitate treatment. Because reason is pure, or innocent, as some contemporary writers claim, the value of rationality is seldom questioned (Murphy, 1989). What reasonable person, in short, attacks rationality?

REASON AND DUALISM

Nonetheless, a host of contemporary critics has challenged the basic assumption of reason. That is, they contend that reason is not pristine; they claim rationality is implicated in the same factors that restrict other approaches to knowledge acquisition and practice. The rationale for this criticism is predicated on their rejection of dualism. The dualism that provides reason with its credibility and unique stature is viewed by these writers to be passé. Michel Foucault, Jacques Derrida, and Jean-Francois Lyotard, for example, advance a theory of language that undermines dualism (Murphy, 1989). While borrowing from the later work of Wittgenstein, they argue that all knowledge is mediated by language use (Murphy, 1989). Every form of knowledge, therefore, is affected by the uncertainty associated with interpretation that reason is supposed to avoid. Because nothing escapes from the effects of language use, reason is tied intimately to the human presence. In the end, to borrow from Foucault (1989), reason is nothing more than a type of discourse.

According to this linguistic thesis, reason exhibits a particular bias. Another way of describing this outcome is to say that rationality is embedded. Indeed, reason is embedded in various epistemological, organizational, and political considerations. The point at this juncture is not to argue that reason is insidious, or untrustworthy, but to acknowledge that rationality is the product of competing definitions and social agendas. Resorting to reason to adjudicate conflicting claims or policies, accordingly, does not guarantee objectivity.

In more concrete terms, science is not value-free, but rather embodies a particular culture. And according to this culture, unique forms of data, search strategies, research methods, and techniques of comparison are treated as normative. Rationality is thus determined by these norms. But, like in any other culture, rules of behavior are not necessarily universal; not recognizing the limits of these norms, accordingly, results in ethnocentrism. Therefore, employing these norms as if they are universal can be very damaging.

The importance of recognizing embeddedness is to encourage social sensitivity. Understanding reason to be a modality of human *praxis* should promote the idea that rationality can take many forms, along with the awareness that objectivity is not automatically guaranteed by science or technology. Because rationality is a cultural theme, the application or study of reason requires social insight that is not objective in the traditional sense.

Reason and Organizational Life

Implied by the notion of embeddedness is that reason is situated in a variety of ways. As Thomas Kuhn (1970) relates, for example, reason is theory-laden; different theoretical discourses can provide reason with divergent meanings. Behaviorists and Structuralists reach very different conclusions about human reasoning and the link between reason and behavior. In this regard, theory is tied intimately to practice.

Similarly, the operation of science and technology is predicated on assumptions about data, calculation, and evaluation. Computer use relies on binary logic, the reduction of knowledge to information bits, and algorithmic instructions to generate output (Dreyfus & Dreyfus, 1986). Reason, accordingly, is little more than reckoning–processing input according to step-wise instructions. Obscured by this approach to reason are the elements necessary for reflection and criticism. Computers, accordingly, cannot address the processes that contribute to the formation and acceptance of data categories. As a result, critics argue that computers simply reify knowledge and the related classificatory activities.

On another level, reason is affected by institutional structures and philosophies. Reason is not the same in a bureaucracy and the more flatly organized workplace. In the former, reason is mechanistic, while in the latter, rationality is less rigid and based on the job to be completed. Furthermore, management style plays a large role in outlining the parameters of reason. Advocates of scientific and humanistic management disagree on the importance of volition in job design. The question is whether or not reason includes the element of unforced choice.

Following the rejection of dualism, reason is tied to practice. And in this discussion, practice refers to both theoretical and very pragmatic concerns. Reason, in this sense, does not provide a picture of reality, but instead is implicated in the various discourses that shape social life. Rather than existing above daily affairs, reason reflects the various projects and activities that persons decide to undertake.

ETHNOCENTRISM AND ORGANIZATIONS

In social science, ethnocentrism is criticized as something to be avoided. Those who are ethnocentric are overtly biased and degrade cultures that are different from their own. Such prejudice is considered to be unfortunate, because scientists are supposed to eschew value judgments. At least, they are supposed to be open-minded enough to appreciate the contribution made by all cultures to civilization.

In order to be accurate, in other words, cultures should be understood in their own terms. To use a term popularized by phenomenologists, researchers should learn to pay attention to the *Lebenswelt*, or "life-world," of persons (Landgrebe, 1966). The life-world consists of a mélange of projects–including the values, beliefs, and commitments–that comprise an organization's history. Within this realm, moreover, are the norms that are invoked to differentiate reality from illusion.

Practitioners should also attempt to gain entry into this experiential domain. Indeed, this sphere holds the key to understanding the discourses that specify the parameters of health and illness. Prescribing an acceptable intervention, accordingly, requires that an organization's mores be properly understood. Without recognizing the influence of the life-world, assessments and treatments are haphazard; these facets of service delivery are undertaken according to ideals that may have no cultural relevance.

Contrary to what might be expected, reason may encourage ethnocentrism. Specifically, because reason is usually touted to be pristine and universal, the reflection that is required to be culturally sensitive is obscured. In fact, reflection is viewed to be subjective, unpredictable, and a source of error. For accuracy to prevail, reason has to be discovered and implemented without any interference from interpretation and similar sources of uncertainty. Reason, in short, shields persons from the problems that arise from human foibles, such as bias, impatience, and lapses of concentration.

But as mentioned earlier, reason is not pure; reason is revealed through various language games. Reason is thus a mode of *praxis* that is concealed behind a façade of universality (Gilroy, 1993). The trouble is that because of this subterfuge, reason is seldom associated with prejudice and partisanism. Nonetheless, according to Stanley Fish (1989), the implementation of reason requires that one form of discourse be allowed to dominate all others. In this regard, ideology hides behind claims made about rationality. Therefore, applying reason does not necessarily result in the clarification of an issue. Overlooked by this strategy are the discourses, ploys, and politics involved in defining truth, giving legitimacy to facts, or differentiating logic from irrationality. The only way in which these issues can be addressed is by consulting the life-world. By entering this realm properly, these processes can be revealed, thereby delineating reason and illustrating the most propitious use of rationality. In a manner of speaking, reason is thus resurrected from a sphere that is often believed to be pervaded by irrationality.

ARTICLE SUMMARIES

These articles grew out of a conference held at Wake Forest University in 1996 entitled "Symposium on Social Dimensions of Rationality and Risk Assessment." This meeting approached the philosophical basis of risk and rationality, especially as applied to medicine and public health issues. Selected papers from that conference, along with others chosen to fill out the picture, are assembled here.

In the first article, "Reason, the Life-World, and Health Care Delivery," Choi and Murphy set the stage with their discussion of the roots of rationality in Western thought. They do not argue that reason and rationality are bad in themselves. They are not. A cultural problem, however, has arisen. Many thinkers, whose concerns are primarily mechanical and technological, claim that rationality must be value-neutral and universal. This is an ethnocentric assertion that claims universality for a particular, mechanistic, view of rationality. Furthermore, this version of reason is ineffective because it is not grounded in the messy and inexact life-worlds of patients, clients, customers and ordinary persons, thereby rendering reason inadequate as a mode of interpretation.

Pardeck, in the second article, "Rationalizing Decision-Making Through Computer Technology," illustrates many of the ideas developed by Choi and Murphy in the context of the computerization of professional decision-making. If reason is value-neutral and universal, then a logical application is computer-based decision-making. Such attempts, unfortunately, have failed because of the impossibility of producing completely unambiguous and consistently meaningful data on which to build such a system. Therefore, professionals who rely on computer-based expert systems must "buy into" them as an act of faith. In other words, the person who believes in rationality's purity and power, as applied to human decision-making, must enter a state described by Samuel Taylor Coleridge as a "willing suspension of disbelief."

Two articles discuss reason and rationality in the context of public health issues. In "Sociomedical Models and the Epistemology of Risk," Vernberg explains several theoretical models of popular decision-making as they apply to health education. These models offer different perspectives on how to encourage individuals to make decisions that are good for their own health. Each model is attached to assumptions and generates policy preferences. For example, the view of rationality in behaviorism promotes the essential inertness and reactivity of humans. That is, individual behavior is seen as being caused entirely by outside forces that can be measured and predicted. Value expectancy models, on the other hand, are based on Bayesian principles, which tend to view rationality as estimates of utility expressed in terms of risk. Such views are commonly found in economic theories that are essentially utilitarian in nature. However, they cannot explain self-destructive behavior or altruism. Third, information processing models are essentially computer models, assuming a bounded rationality within which choices are made among known alternatives in order to maximize outcomes. Finally, Vernberg recommends the empowerment model, which is consistent with a phenomenological understanding of intentionality. This model offers a view of rationality that is hopeful in that it grounds perceptions in the practical contexts that enliven motivation and move the human will to action.

Smith argues in the fourth article, "Community-Based Epidemiology: Community Involvement in Defining Social Risk," that traditional understandings of rationality have focused epidemiological research on individual risk factors that can be individually modified. Unfortunately, this approach misses the essential complexity and connectedness of health issues. Community-based epidemiology, on the other hand, partners the researcher and the community in such a way that the context and meaning of the community can help define research issues, interpret findings, and propose outcomes, thereby increasing the effectiveness of resulting solutions to health problems. Consistent with Vernberg's discussion, empowerment, once again, has a central place in the process.

The final three articles focus on aspects of the lived experience of patients, providers and organizations, all in the setting of biomedicine. Each, in its own way, argues that rationality cannot be universal and value-neutral, but is seen as very contextual.

In the fifth article, "A World View Model of Health Care Utilization: The Impact of Social and Provider Context on Health Care Decision-Making," Daley and Bostock picture health care as a dance between consumers and providers. Each brings its own reality to the encounter. Reason, thus, is the negotiation of different worldviews to produce an outcome. Daley and Bostock show that rationality is perhaps less a thing than a process, not reason, but reasoning. Symptoms must be interpreted. Otherwise, health care would not be sought. The individual interprets symptoms through several filters, for example, through the meaning given the symptom by her family and social network. Health care resources also are brought to the meeting. Like symptoms, these resources are also filtered through the provider and, in the case of managed care, the providing organization. The result of the encounter, perhaps, is a diagnosis and a treatment plan. In this scenario, rationality is consensus, an outcome of reasoning, in which the provider convinces the consumer of the diagnosis and in which the consumer agrees to the treatment plan. The empowerment of both parties is implied in such an outcome.

In the sixth article, "Health Care Policy in Theory and Practice," Prosono describes another kind of negotiation, the interaction between political and organizational environments and health care policy. Each paper in this collection argues that rationality is not something pristine and ethereal, standing apart from the life-worlds of humans. Prosono comes close to arguing, in this paper, that there is a counterpart to the life-world that operates for occupational and political cultures, and that health policy must be negotiated, just as rationality itself is negotiated. Four historical turning points in health care policy are discussed contextually. The Medical Police concept succeeded in Germany at the end of the eighteenth century, establishing the citizen's right to health care, and the right of the government to police health care. At the turn of the twentieth century, organized medicine was reformed in the United States, swept along by the legitimating power of science. The Flexner Report is a useful metaphor for the transformation. In 1946, the Hill Burton Act, to expand hospital construction in the United States, was pushed by a diverse coalition of interests, satisfying important positions of both liberals and conservatives. On the other hand, the Clinton Plan, in 1994, failed because it essentially ignored its political and organizational contexts. Like the notion of pure reason, the aloofness of the process was fatal.

In the final article by Longino, "The Limits of Scientific Medicine: Paradigm Strain and Social Policy," the argument is made that biomedicine is rooted philosophically in a long philosophical tradition. These philosophical roots keep biomedicine focused on the body and away from the connections between mind and body and the social and cultural contexts of the body. The worldview was consolidated under pressure to find cures for acute diseases. The Cartesian paradigm has been increasingly strained, however, by the prevalence and eventual domination of chronic diseases. Again, rather than looking for linear causal connections within the body that point to a "magic bullet" solution, the emerging paradigm must be much more contextual and less reductionistic to fit the current and future understanding of health.

These seven articles, taken together, provide a phenomenological critique of pure rationality in biomedicine and health care today. Once again, rationality, per se, is not to be eschewed. The understanding of reason, however, must be much better grounded in the life-world, and social contexts, so that the outcomes generated by reason can be effective.

REFERENCES

Dreyfus, H. L. & Dreyfus, S. E. (1986). *Mind over machine*. NY: The Free Press.
Fish, S. (1989). *Doing what comes naturally*. Durham, NC: Duke University Press.
Foucault, M. (1989). *The archaeology of knowledge*. London: Routledge.
Gilroy, P. (1993). *The black Atlantic*. London: Verso.
Kuhn, T. S. (1970). *The structure of scientific revolutions*. Chicago: University of Chicago Press.
Landgrebe, L. (1966). *Major problems in contemporary European philosophy*. NY: Frederick Unger.
Longino, C. F. & Murphy, J. W. (1995). *The old-age challenge to the biomedical model*. Amityville, NY: Baywood.
Murphy, J. W. (1989). *Postmodernism social analysis and criticism*. Westport, CT: Greenwood.

Reason, the Life-World, and Health Care Delivery

Jung Min Choi, PhD
John W. Murphy, PhD

SUMMARY. Reason is illustrated to be conceived traditionally in an abstract manner. The attempt has been made to make rationality appear value-neutral and universal. In the end, however, this version of reason is ineffective, because the human element is overlooked. Contemporary philosophy is shown to have abandoned this ethereal view of knowledge and reason. Furthermore, interventions that are based on this shift in theory are more socially sensitive and appropriate. *[Article copies available for a fee from The Haworth Document Delivery Service: 1-800-342-9678. E-mail address: getinfo@haworth.com]*

ABSTRACT REASON

At the core of Western intellectual life is foundationalism. This designation, write postmodernists, means that "metanarratives" have been sought to sustain knowledge and order (Lyotard, 1984, p. xxiv). These Grand Narratives, as they are sometimes called, represent explanations for identity, social institutions, and laws that are not embroiled in quotidian concerns. Because of these absolutes, ethical claims and behavioral standards are thought to have an inviolable justification.

Jung Min Choi is Assistant Professor of Sociology, Barry University, Miami Shores, FL 33161. John W. Murphy is Professor of Sociology, University of Miami, Coral Gables, FL 33124.

[Haworth co-indexing entry note]: "Reason, the Life-World, and Health Care Delivery." Choi, Jung Min, and John W. Murphy. Co-published simultaneously in *Journal of Health & Social Policy* (The Haworth Press, Inc.) Vol. 9, No. 4, 1998, pp. 9-17; and: *Reason and Rationality in Health and Human Services Delivery* (ed: John T. Pardeck, Charles F. Longino, Jr., and John W. Murphy) The Haworth Press, Inc., 1998, pp. 9-17. Single or multiple copies of this article are available for a fee from The Haworth Document Delivery Service [1-800-342-9678, 9:00 a.m. - 5:00 p.m. (EST). E-mail address: getinfo@haworth.com].

Assumed by foundationalism is a mode of thinking that achieved notoriety circa 1600. In general, this outlook is referred to as dualism. Foundationalists are dualistic because their aim is to ground knowledge and order on an ahistorical principle. In other words, escape from the everyday realm of interpretation, opinion, and contingency is not only possible, but is encouraged. Descartes formalized this claim when he declared that *res cogitans* should be separated categorically from *res extensa* (Stumpf, 1975). As a result of this demarche, a foundation that is untrammeled by situational exigencies can be invoked to verify all judgements. A referent for truth is available that is severed from opinion, because interpretation is unrelated to the validity of knowledge claims.

Reason has not been exempt from this trend. As a central factor in the acquisition of knowledge and the preservation of both natural and social harmony, reason has been given a unique status. Reason could not be contaminated by interpretation; rationality could not be linked to considerations that may bias decision-making. In order to be accurate and reliable, reason has to be pure and precise. Therefore, any factor that might compromise the exercise of reason had to be discarded, or rationality would not be automatically universal.

The early Greeks understood reason to be an all-encompassing cosmic principle (Murphy, 1989). Thales invoked water, while Pythagoras introduced Number to explain the natural order of events. For Heraclitus, Logos supplied the rationale for the harmony that prevails in both nature and society. The key point is that an eternal steering mechanism is presumed to guide personal actions and sustain the relationships found in nature.

Later on, a similar theme is found in the work of Plato and Aristotle, although their foundations are thought to be slightly less esoteric than earlier writers. As Plato discussed in his *Republic,* escape from daily existence is essential to achieve wisdom. Once entree is gained to the sphere occupied by the Forms, the secrets of life are revealed; the order indigenous to the mind, nature, and society becomes clear. These basic and universal archetypes illustrate the inherent identities of persons and objects, in addition to the rules for analyzing correctly natural or social events.

Plato's strategy for insuring the correctness of thinking is made more concrete by Aristotle. Aristotle introduced the syllogism, which would gradually become synonymous with logic. In fact, he contends the syllogism guarantees that conclusions follow properly from premises. For example, if A > B, and B > C, then A > C. But fundamental to this sequence, however, is the identity of A. Accordingly, Aristotle interjected primordial categories instead of Forms to insure that A is unambiguous. These frames supply the essential traits of A, so that A can never be confused with B, C, or any other entity. In the end, Aristotle's categories perform a function identical to Plato's Forms, for in each case rationality is provided with an indubitable framework.

During the Medieval Period, the source of reason was transformed into something overtly ethereal. Insight into God's creations was thought to offer clues pertaining to the character of reason. According to St. Thomas Aquinas, perusing nature illustrates the basic rationality of the natural world, which, in turn, provides evidence for the existence of God. This entire process, however, is replete with speculation and elements of mysticism.

The Renaissance provided a break from these sorts of cosmic questions, without abandoning hope of discovering reason. Through observation and empirical research, rather than unprincipled illumination, the laws of reason can be exposed. As a result of rigorous experimentation, and using recently developed technical instruments, the basic properties and causal relationships present in the universe can be understood by everyone.

Descartes reinforced this viewpoint by declaring that clear and distinct knowledge can be acquired by sequestering objectivity from subjectivity (Bordo, 1987). He assumed not only that this distinction is legitimate, but that once subjectivity is controlled, true knowledge is readily accessible. This Cartesian dualism, accordingly, reinforced the use of scientific instruments. Scientific devices, in short, are touted to be the neutral conduits that enable persons to confront objective knowledge, without any interference from interpretation (Ackerman, 1985).

Through the use of science, the Western dream of catching a glimpse of eternal truth remains alive. Yet, at this historical juncture, this vision is not achieved through esoteric beliefs or practices. Rather, reason is revealed and mastered through sophisticated calculation and methodological refinements. Reason, similar to any other phenomenon, can be described and developed into a formal system. When stabilized in this way, reason can be extended almost indefinitely; only procedural flaws, which have technical remedies, are presumed to restrict the application of reason.

TECHNOLOGY AND MODERN DECISION-MAKING

Subsequent to Descartes' proclamations, the acquisition of knowledge became a mechanical affair. Consistent with his appraisal of dualism, objectivity was transformed into sense data, while subjectivity was referred to as a blank slate. And in the fashion envisioned by empiricists, knowledge is gained when sense impressions are imprinted on the mind. Through a series of cause and effect relationships, the mind and reality are aligned; subjectivity and objectivity are thus joined without blurring the distinction between these two realms.

Considering this desire to deanimate (i.e., neutralize the presence of the human element) the process of gathering information, the activity of the mind was also formalized. Also around 1600, Hobbes argued that mental activity, or reasoning, consisted of what he called reckoning (Dreyfus and Dreyfus, 1982). According to this portrayal of the mind, individualized packets of information are introduced into the mind and classified in a discrete manner. Reasoning thus became equated with the ability to record the objective features of this input in a systematic way, and to make reasonable judgements based on the resulting empirical patterns.

Later, philosophers such as Pascal and Leibnitz, along with Boole, Babbage, and other mathematicians, refined this imagery. With their assistance, the mind was transformed into a logic machine. There, through the operation of a myriad of switches, input is organized in a binary manner. Bits of information are treated as 1's or 0's and processed. The specific arrangement of 1's and 0's determines the message that is received, in addition to the behavior that is expected. In this regard, aligning inputs and outputs with consistency is essential to reasoning.

For the most part, the field of Artificial Intelligence (AI) has been predicated on this rendition of the mind (Murphy and Pardeck, 1991). True to foundationalism, an idealized, or ahistorical, image of mental activity has been adopted. In short, contextless pieces of information trip mechanical switches, thereby forming messages that are unadulterated by interpretation. As a result, analysis and decision-making are possible that are exact and consistent. Because of this precision, the organization and use of knowledge are undertaken in a way the early Greeks could never have imagined.

For the past thirty years, advocates of AI have tried to computerize reason. Given the formalized approach that has been recommended to conceptualizing the mind, linking the computer to cognition was not initially considered to be difficult. After all, in both cases, binary logic is employed to catalogue input; a body of objective knowledge is thus produced that can be used to assess future events (Heim, 1993). And many routine tasks have been successfully computerized, because they can be dissected and operationalized without any loss of meaning.

In the delivery of human services, expert systems have become quite popular. These devices are computer programs that are designed to mimic and, eventually, replace experts. Efficiency and effectiveness are thought to be improved because the human element, which is presumed to be the source of most errors, is removed from any task that is thoroughly computerized. These programs never have a bad day, and therefore this technology is considered to be more reliable than human experts. For example, expert programs are available that can monitor case records, assess clients, and even conduct therapy. In some circles, these applications of computers are thought to enhance service delivery, because the decisions that guide an intervention are allegedly unaffected by emotion, prior experiences, or other sources of bias (Hudson, Nurius, and Reisman, 1988).

What could be more rational than a machine that simply follows instructions without any equivocation? As Dreyfus and Dreyfus (1986) point out, however, these systems are unable to perform like experts. Contrary to this technology, human experts are sensitive to the context of behavior, know when the usual rules of reason do not apply, and can improvise to solve problems. To borrow from Terry Winograd's critique of expert systems, the logic adopted by human experts is not as brittle or rigid as the form of reason that is used in these devices (Dreyfus and Dreyfus, 1986). Stated differently, expert systems operate in terms of a contrived environment, where social, cultural, and other interpretive considerations are assumed to be impediments to sound reasoning. But, throughout most of Western philosophy, this differentiation has been accepted as vital to securing truth.

RATIONALITY AND THE LIFE-WORLD

Much of the philosophy in Europe after WW II represented an attack on dualism. Phenomenology, existentialism, and many approaches to Marxism rejected the idea that true knowledge resides in a sphere sequestered from opinion. A few positivists and empiricists were still visible, but most critics were no longer fascinated by the prospect of discovering the universal laws of either society or nature. The human presence could not be ignored; even physicists recognized that the human project pervades whatever is studied. In Sartrean language, existence precedes essence, because human action is a prerequisite of any rendition of truth (Sartre, 1947).

Lyotard makes this point recently by relying on the later work of Wittgenstein. Lyotard's (1984) claim is that all knowledge, even that associated with science, is mediated completely by "language games" (pp. 9-11). As a result, there is no escape from the circle of interpretation. Attempting to discover Platonic or Aristotelian ideals, for example, is futile, because all knowledge must be formulated within the domain of interpretation that was formerly eschewed. Knowledge and interpretation, simply put, are inextricably linked.

Because of this challenge to dualism, foundationalism loses legitimacy. There is no Archimedean point that provides a neutral or unbiased view of reality. Because of the ubiquity of interpretation, every truth embodies a perspective; every truth can thus be contested and reformulated. Different discursive formations, writes Foucault (1989), allow truth to be reconstructed in a variety of ways. Nonetheless, reliable knowledge does not disappear, but only absolutes devoid of a context are considered to be dubious. Rules exist within each interpretive framework that differentiate reality from illusion; without a humanly constructed context, however, nothing is revealed.

Because of this inability to escape from interpretation, phenomenologists have argued a new approach is needed to describe the origin of knowledge. In the absence of dualism, all knowledge must emerge from the Lebenswelt or life-world. The life-world is the interpretive horizon that persons occupy, which is replete with values, beliefs, and commitments; the life-world is the cultural milieu created by human *praxis* (Husserl, 1970).

The upshot of this theoretical maneuver is that the meaning of facts is socially created, along with the criteria for truth. Therefore, as Lyotard (1984) notes, norms are "locally determined" and reflect shifts in interpretation. And as might be expected, reason is no longer pristine and presumed to reflect universal categories and principles.

As is depicted by Alfred Schutz (1962), the life-world is comprised of multiple realities, and each of these regions represents a legitimate modality of interpretation. The version of reality constructed by science, for example, exists alongside others. Although one of these regions may gain dominance, this exalted position is not secure. As a consequence of changing interpretations, or shifting political alliances, reality may acquire a new cast. Another interpretive region may come to be known as the "so-called" paramount reality, similar to the status currently allotted to science. Indeed, within the life-world these alterations are continuous.

EMBODIED ACTION

Grounded within the life-world, reason is understood to be embodied. The thrust of this new designation is to suggest that reason is not boundless; instead, rationality has parameters and a context. These dimensions, moreover, are an outgrowth of *praxis* and are not arranged in any predetermined manner. Because interpretation extends simultaneously in a number of directions, no categories of rationality are superior inherently to any others. Interpretations do not have the stature required to command this type of recognition.

All possible modes of rationality are juxtaposed to one another, with some periodically elevated in importance. There is no natural continuum or hierarchy of reason, in other words, with all forms of rationality ordered with respect to their purity. As compared to a hierarchy, a lattice work provides a more accurate portrayal of how the numerous modes of reason are related. Because the life-world is crisscrossed by interpretation, any nexus of language games can serve as the basis of rationality.

Rather than abstract, reason is embedded within interpretation. A proper understanding of decision-making, therefore, requires that entree be gained to the operative language game. Appreciating why a particular conclusion has been reached, or a particular behavioral option has been chosen, requires that a specific region of rationality be entered. Hence, as Stanley Fish (1989) is fond of saying, reason is political rather than neutral. The explanatory power of reason is operative, in other words, only after primacy has been given to a specific domain of rationality; reason comes into play only subsequent to giving credence to one of many language games. In this regard, the foundation of reason is imbued with volition and thoroughly historical.

GROUNDED INTERVENTION

Clearly, this change in viewing reason has relevance for planning interventions. Methodological precision and logistical rigor are no longer sufficient to improve the delivery of health services. Using abstract formulas, although ones that may be considered to be formalized and objective, will not necessarily increase the relevance or utility of an intervention. What will likely be overlooked is the actual social setting, thus making planning increasingly haphazard. The search for objectivity, in this case, is counterproductive; instead of avoided, bias that is based in science is allowed to obscure social life.

In order for interventions to become more accurate, the usual sources of inaccuracy must be explored. As suggested by Glazer and Strauss (1967), interventions must become more grounded. Specifically, the connection that exists between interpretation and reason should be investigated. The attempt has been made traditionally to separate these two considerations, but now appreciating the link between them is crucial to a successful intervention.

According to Weber (1978) truth is based more on interpretive adequacy than a tightly formulated system of logic. What he means is that a mastery of important axioms does not guarantee the development of a socially relevant understanding of behavior. In this case, an accurate intervention is not necessarily an outgrowth of formalized propositions. The rationale for this conclusion is quite simple: logical arguments may be internally consistent, but may begin in the wrong place. The usual correction for this problem is to make sure that logic reflects reality. But subsequent to the recent challenge to dualism, this gambit is impossible. Accordingly, a logical argument must be verified by consulting the relevant language game, because the usual universals are occluded by interpretation.

Whether reasoning is true or false depends on how closely a mode of logic is related to a specific interpretive domain. A close association, for example, increases the legitimacy of a particular form of reason. The degree of this linkage is what Weber refers to as interpretive adequacy. Instead of unbiased, the best reason is properly biased; the reason with the most explanatory power is tied the closest to daily existence. Sound reasoning, in other words, is predicated on interpretation rather than ideals of logic.

Rather than acuity at logic, "communicative competence" is most important for an intervention to be successful (Habermas, 1970). This skill, moreover, is not a product of logical precision, methodological rigor, or technical refinement. In fact, these practices may actually induce error, because their aim is to escape from any influence exerted by the human presence. Engaging a client's or community's life-world—most important, the relevant interpretive base of reality—is not a part of this agenda.

Communicative competence is achieved by addressing the language game that underpins reason. Grasping the pragmatic thrust of the relevant language game is essential to gaining insight to any system of logic. And because the fundamental categories of any mode of logic are socially invented, and thus do not exist *sui generis,* dialogue is vital to creating an appropriate intervention. Contrary to what has been usually accepted, subjectivity is at the core of accuracy; interpretation is at the center of an unbiased assessment. Specifically, entering the life-world of those to be serviced, through discourse with the appropriate community, is necessary to make an intervention socially sensitive and, thus, rational.

Elements that have been assumed to be antithetical to rationality are now important for sustaining the rationale that guides an intervention. Values, beliefs, and a host of other situational contingencies or interpretive relevancies should not be ignored when attempting to intervene rationally into social affairs. Practitioners should not be distracted from these considerations by the lure of formal rationality and claims about the fruits of science. In fact, failure to review these factors will result, most likely, in purely rational, but irrelevant correctives. This kind of misunderstanding may spawn serious and costly mistakes.

REFERENCES

Ackerman, R.J. (1985). *Data, instruments, and theory.* Princeton, NJ: Princeton University Press.
Bordo, S. (1987). *The flight to objectivity.* Albany: SUNY Press.
Dreyfus, H.L. & Dreyfus, S.E. (1986). *Mind over machine.* NY: The Free Press.
Fish, S. (1989). *Doing what comes naturally.* Durham: Duke University Press.
Foucault, M. (1989). *The archaeology of knowledge.* London: Routledge.
Glaser, B.G. & Strauss, A.L. (1967). *The discovery of grounded theory.* Chicago: Aldine.
Habermas, J. (1970). Toward a theory of communicative competence. In H.P. Dreitzel (Ed.), *Recent sociology,* No. 2 (pp. 115-148). NY: Macmillan.
Heim, M. (1993). *The metaphysics of virtual reality.* NY: Oxford University Press.
Hudson, W.W., Nurius, P.A. & Reisman, S. (1988). Computerized assessment instruments: Their promises and problems. In J.W. Murphy & J.T. Pardeck (Eds.), *Technology and human service delivery* (pp. 51-70). NY: The Haworth Press, Inc.
Husserl, E. (1970). *The crisis of European sciences and transcendental pheno-menology.* Evanston: Northwestern University Press.
Lyotard, J-F. (1984). *The postmodern condition.* Minneapolis: University of Minnesota Press.
Murphy, J.W. (1989). *Postmodern social analysis and criticism.* Westport, CT: Greenwood.
Murphy, J.W. & Pardeck, J.T. (1991). *The computerization of human service agencies.* NY: Auburn House.
Sartre, J-P. (1947). *Existentialism.* NY: The Philosophical Library.
Schutz, A. (1962). *Collected papers.* Vol I. The Hague: Nijhoff.
Stumpf, S.E. (1975). *Socrates to Sartre.* NY: McGraw-Hill.
Weber, M. (1978). *Economy and society.* Vol. I. Berkeley: University of California Press.

Rationalizing Decision-Making Through Computer Technology: A Critical Appraisal

John T. Pardeck, PhD, ACSW

SUMMARY. As human services become more complex and multi-faceted, sound decision-making guiding the service delivery process becomes critical. Administrators and others view computer technology as a means to rationalize the decision-making process at all levels of organizational life. The Management Information System (MIS) and program evaluations are viewed as technologies particularly useful for enhancing the decision-making process through computer technology. The strengths and limitations of computer technology are discussed. Strategies for using computer technology responsibly are offered. *[Article copies available for a fee from The Haworth Document Delivery Service: 1-800-342-9678. E-mail address: getinfo@haworth.com]*

Human service agencies are increasingly becoming more complex and multifaceted as they respond to the changing needs of society. Computer technology is seen by many administrators as a means for meeting the challenges that change brings. Computerization is viewed as a strategy that will enhance human services functioning through the rationalization of the decision-making process at all levels of organizational life (Pardeck, in press).

John T. Pardeck is Professor of Social Work, School of Social Work at Southwest Missouri State University, Springfield, MO 65804.

[Haworth co-indexing entry note]: "Rationalizing Decision-Making Through Computer Technology: A Critical Appraisal." Pardeck, John T. Co-published simultaneously in *Journal of Health & Social Policy* (The Haworth Press, Inc.) Vol. 9, No. 4, 1998, pp. 19-29; and: *Reason and Rationality in Health and Human Services Delivery* (ed: John T. Pardeck, Charles F. Longino, Jr., and John W. Murphy) The Haworth Press, Inc., 1998, pp. 19-29. Single or multiple copies of this article are available for a fee from The Haworth Document Delivery Service [1-800-342-9678, 9:00 a.m. - 5:00 p.m. (EST). E-mail address: getinfo@haworth.com].

19

Computer technology demands that all aspects of the human services agency must be translated into the language of computers. This means that virtually any aspect of organizational life must be quantitative. Quantification of practice activities results in all aspects of treatment being conceptualized in concrete terms. Obviously, certain aspects of social treatment do not lend themselves well to computerization; these behaviors must be eliminated or conducted in the traditional fashion. However, the nonquantifiable aspect of social intervention may not be recorded by practitioners in the clinical record. Thus, a large percentage of service delivery may never be recorded or understood by those concerned with the accountability of the practitioner's performance (Murphy & Pardeck, 1991).

It is not uncommon for practitioners to reject the notion that practice can be quantified. Central to this argument is that the helping process is so abstract that many treatment interventions cannot be quantified or translated into the language of computers. However, this form of rationalization of the treatment process is demanded by computer technology; treatment must be reduced to the logic of computerization (Boden, 1977).

A MICROCOMPUTER SYSTEM

Microcomputers are the most popular technology used to rationalize organizational activities. Administrators feel that this technology will enhance organizational efficiency and decision-making. Microcomputer technology also allows workers to be linked to one another. This linkage allows workers to communicate with one another through their individual microcomputers.

The storage medium for the microcomputer is usually the disk. However, many users are beginning to store information on cartridges. This technology allows the user to store an infinite amount of information. The many software packages available help the user perform countless activities which support the work process. The microcomputer can facilitate many organizational activities. These are typically as follows: inventory testing, word processing, and recording (Murphy & Pardeck, 1991).

Inventory Testing

Software packages are now available that can assess the presenting problem of clients. For example, the Minnesota Multiphasic Personality Inventory (MMPI) can be administered and scored via a microcomputer. Practitioners may doubt the validity of this procedure, yet users routinely report that clients often prefer automated testing over the paper-and-pencil administered inventory. Since the processing of inventories is automated, scales can be scored accurately and rapidly, resulting in instant feedback to the client and practitioner.

Word Processing

There are many software packages available to practitioners that enable them to create and edit documents, in addition to printing them. This technology allows for improved record keeping, as case records can be neatly recorded, easily stored, and put in a standardized format. Other uses for word processing are for letter writing and reports.

Advanced editing and typing functions, such as corrections, centering, insertions, and deletions, may be performed with several simple key strokes. The advantage of word processing is that a client's progress can be documented on disk or other storage devices, resulting in treatment plans and management reports being generated with little effort when needed. Word processing clearly facilitates many basic organizational and clinical activities.

Recording

Documenting, monitoring, and recording assessment activities are critical to the treatment process. Programs are available that can conduct the psychosocial interview and record the results of this clinical process. Automated interviews, as they are sometimes called, follow a fixed format protocol, and thus have been evaluated by some as more comprehensive than open-ended or free-flowing approaches. During an intake interview, pressures are often present that result in practitioners forgetting information or not asking particular questions. This type of format, utilized by computerized interviews, which assists in monitoring, documenting, and recording information is designed to prevent these types of omissions, which can make a record sloppy and inaccurate.

If many clients are being served, the reviewing of treatment plans can be very time consuming and difficult to organize. Treatment plans based on goal attainment scaling, for example, can be easily computerized, since specific treatment objectives must be precisely defined in measurable terms. A timetable can be developed which indicates when a plan needs to be reviewed next. In addition to treatment plans, software packages have been developed for standardizing medical and counseling records. The result of these applications requires that information be conceptualized clearly and precisely, thereby allowing the fixed-format classification to be implemented.

MANAGEMENT INFORMATION SYSTEM (MIS)

The 1990s can be viewed as the decade of computer technology (Murphy & Pardeck, 1991). Political and social events have necessitated the establishment of the computerized human services agencies. This technological strategy allows agencies to use computer technology in planning and delivery of services, their subsequent evaluation, and fiscal support. Furthermore, status indicators of the human services agency have changed since the 1970s and 1980s. For example, to have psychiatric consultation readily available in the agency was an important status symbol. Often, status is determined by the number of computers and the amount of data collected. Moreover, many agencies are collecting data without adequate conceptual rationale, thus reducing its relevance for human services programming (Karger & Kreuger, 1988).

The MIS is the core strategy currently used to computerize the majority of agency functions. Information systems compatibility is key to design and functionality. For example, if an information system is being installed in a mental health agency, it is critical that it be compatible with the other agencies providing key services to clients being served. One way to accomplish this goal is to have yearly evaluations of information being collected and exchanged between agencies. This evaluation should address how other human services professionals use the information, the types of data collected, and how the organization is designed to facilitate the use of the data.

The following kinds of questions should be asked when developing an MIS: What type of data is needed? What kind of software is required? What forms will be required to collect the data? and How will the data be stored? If there are tremendous differences between information systems, service delivery will break down, thus having negative consequences for clients.

Core data collected by the agency should focus on clients, workers and treatment outcomes, and processes critical to service delivery. These data allow managers to see how clients are served, what workers provide them, and the kinds and length of treatment being implemented. This critical information allows agencies to conduct other important activities essential to the accountability process such as cost-benefit analysis. In terms of social treatment, an MIS provides invaluable data regarding client assessment, evaluations of services, documentation of interventions and treatment follow-up.

When designing an MIS system, files are normally in free-form or fixed-form format. Free-form can be used to record client assessment, treatment, and follow-up. They allow personnel to describe clinical activities in great detail; however, they are difficult to summarize and condense.

The fixed-form format record specifies the exact data to be collected by the worker. This may be in a structured interview schedule used to secure descriptive data on clients. The computer can quickly summarize the number of clients served, their ages, income, marital status and other important information. Obviously, the qualitative component of treatment does not easily translate into the fixed-format record.

Before an agency implements an MIS, all organizational personnel should be involved in its development. This participation should help build understanding of the system and help to minimize opposition to its implementation. Murphy and Pardeck (1991) suggest the following non-technical issues must be considered for successful development of an MIS:

1. Understand clearly the management philosophy.
2. Identify key decision-makers and the types of decisions that will have to be made.
3. Locate vital sources of information, and determine the most appropriate ways to gather this data.
4. Calculate the amount of effort needed to garner relevant information in a socially sensitive manner.
5. Attempt to integrate conceptual, logistical and social considerations.
6. Determine the social character of relevant data.
7. Know the culture of an organization, so that the information will flow smoothly from place to place.
8. Appreciate how the conceptual side of MIS development can enhance research and other activities.
9. Use an MIS project as an opportunity to integrate an organization.

It should be noted that there are no shortcuts to properly developing an MIS. Agencies should not rush into the process and should consider not only the technical side of development but also the non-technical components.

As should be obvious, the managerial applications of an MIS are extensive. A major area of application for management in the delivery of services is that of information management. Management has found that computer technology can be a tremendous time saver in compiling reports and payrolls. Computer technology now allows agencies to conduct advanced program evaluations for analyzing agency activities that were simply impossible in the past (Dreyfus & Dreyfus, 1986). As management and workers realize, an inordinate amount of time and energy in traditional human service agencies is devoted to paperwork. An MIS can dramatically reduce paperwork generation through producing and storing data in the computerized information system rather than storing it on paper. This approach is far more cost effective and efficient for storing data. An efficient MIS system can facilitate the agency's billing, financial screening procedures, review and revision of fee schedules, and maintenance of accurate accounts of operating reserves to reduce cash flow problems (Schoech, 1992).

Program Evaluation

Modern day computer technology has revolutionized how agencies conduct research and conduct program evaluations. A few decades ago, computer applications in human services were extremely limited and were largely used for only accounting and bureaucratic record keeping. The microcomputer, in particular, has allowed agencies to conduct numerous kinds of evaluation efficiently and effectively (Pardeck, Murphy, & Callaghan, 1994).

The traditional use of the computer in program evaluation has been to assist in coding and analyzing data. Microcomputer software packages are available that allow agency personnel to conduct advanced statistical analyses such as multiple regression and factor analysis. In the past, this kind of advanced multivariate statistical analysis could only be conducted by a mainframe computer system. Other software packages available to human services agencies can help select a sample for data analysis as well as other related research activities.

Other important research capabilities of present day computer technology are that it can assist in literature review, create spreadsheets, and provide graphic displays such as charts and figures which help to communicate the findings of research and program evaluation.

Outcome Measures

Program evaluation calls for the measurement of treatment outcome. In the past, formal assessments were largely paper-and-pencil devices that were completed by the client and scored by the practitioner. Numerous clinical scales have been computerized. Having scales in a computerized format means they can easily be used in assessment and in the measurement of treatment outcome (Stuart, 1988).

The computerized interview is another development which not only facilitates the intervention process but also clearly assists practitioners in evaluation of treatment outcome. The computerized interview is highly standardized in format, and is extremely reliable. Erdman and Foster (1988) conclude, in contrast to human-administered interviews, that computer interviews are 100% reliable; computers never forget to ask a question, and given the same pattern of responses by a client, the computer will always ask the same questions in the same way. Such standardization allows for comparison between clinical cases, which can improve on the traditional strategies used for evaluating treatment outcome.

Collecting sensitive information from clients may be easier through the use of computers. Clients will be more apt to provide a computer with sensitive information versus telling a human being. Colby (1980) summarized the advantages of the computer over the human being:

It [the computer] does not get tired, angry, or bored. It is always willing to listen and to give evidence of being heard. It can work at any time of the day or night, every day of the week, every month of the year. It does not have family problems of its own. It never gets sick or hung over. Its performance does not vary from hour to hour or from day to day. (p. 14)

Colby's remarks would suggest the reliability of the research process is enhanced. Furthermore, computer administered questions can increase data integrity by virtually eliminating incomplete responses since it calls the client's attention to items not completed. As most individuals involved in program evaluation and other forms of social research realize, the problem of missing data from respondents is a major methodological issue to be dealt with. The computer can eliminate most of this challenge largely caused by human error.

Computers have entered program evaluation in novel ways through new software packages which evaluate the presenting problems of clients and assess treatment progress through direct interaction with the computer. This form of evaluation is based on the single-subject design.

The power of the single-subject design is that it is based on statistical analysis, which in turn helps clinicians decide if a treatment is working or not. The practitioner can simply adopt existing software to implement the single-subject design or select specifically tailored software packages available for data analysis.

There are many software packages available for microcomputers that will quickly provide line graphs, histograms, pie charts, and other visual displays for data. The spreadsheet is one of the most popular. With the spreadsheet, the researcher can graph data and do an array of statistical evaluations. It derives its name from the common accounting system of organizing financial data on special grids of rows and columns known as spreadsheets. Even though accounting applications were the impetus for spreadsheets, practitioners have discovered many different uses of the program; in particular, its application to single-subject evaluation and research.

Clearly computers are essential for research and program evaluation purposes. The development of the microcomputer has allowed agencies to conduct calculations of data that were extremely complicated just two decades ago but are now routine. Transformation of data, graphing of client goals, and modifications of data for further analysis are simple routines for the microcomputer. For example, the frequently used Statistical Package for the Social Sciences (SPSSX) and other statistical packages are now available for use with the microcomputer. This important innovation increases the capability of practitioners to execute basic statistical analyses on their cases.

CONCLUSION

The numerous ways in which computers can enhance service delivery and decision-making have been presented in this paper. However, even though computerization appears to increase the efficiency of an agency, a number of key points must be raised about the implications of this technology on service delivery. These points are built around Luhman's (1982) argument that the more computerized an organization becomes, the less it becomes attuned to the social world. Furthermore, as emphasized by Murphy and Pardeck (1991), even though computerization may create the illusion of objectivity and rationality within the organization, the data collected on clients may not produce useful information for social intervention. In fact, much of it may simply be irrelevant to the workings of the social world of clients and the larger community. Therefore, a number of non-technical factors must receive attention before computerization can enhance the functioning and decision-making processes of the social services agency.

Management Philosophy

Serious attention must be devoted to the management philosophy adhered to by administrators. Computerization of an organization will only work if the logic used by managers to make decisions is known by workers. Computers can be programmed to produce relevant information, thereby enhancing a manager's ability to make sound judgments. Nonetheless, the impact of management philosophy on a person's decision-making ability is often ignored within organizations. Managers, simply put, are assumed to use universally accepted standards when evaluating their options, with minor miscalculations occurring.

Computerization of the organization is theoretically supposed to eliminate these errors. However, a manager's philosophy (e.g., human relations versus Taylorism) determines the type of data that is considered to be important, in addition to how knowledge about an agency should be used.

Goals and Objectives

The goals and objectives of an organization must be understood. Most often, however, this idea is translated to mean that goals should clearly be operationalized. More often than not, the relevance of the goals of an organization to the social world are not shared. In fact, within human service organizations, it is assumed that all of these systems are operating under similar goals–often they are not. Even when the question of goals is raised, the analysis is often irrelevant and narrow. Key decision-makers and funding agencies are consulted to discover what they believe the agency should accomplish, yet seldom are clients, workers, or community members involved directly in planning the delivery of social services. The question must not be dismissed: Who are the "stakeholders" in the agency? Obviously, such a query cannot be answered without transcending the boundary set by the technological ethic, in order to incorporate legal, ethical, economic, and political considerations into what data is collected in an agency; then, in turn, how it is used in service delivery.

The Nature of Data

What are data? Usually this question prompts a response steeped in methodological argument. For example, facts are different than opinions because the former are a product of science. Valid data thus are generated through procedures that are rigorous. Computerization of the human service agency is supposed to help generate sound scientific data. Other forms of information are cited as inaccurate due to the influences of human error. Yet, collection practices are only indirectly related to validity; many businesses are beginning to recognize this point. After the installation of computers, culmination of data collection becomes an end in itself. It should always be emphasized that policy-related questions, such as, how data are used, what type of decisions are to be made, and what are the criteria to be used for decision-making, provide knowledge with its meaning. A unit of service, which is something practitioners often take for granted, may have an entirely different meaning for a client, clinician, federal bureaucrat, or an accountant in a local human services agency. Thus, how data are collected and defined is a key element in the successful computerization of an agency.

Data Collection

A sophisticated data collection apparatus is insufficient to guarantee that information will flow throughout an organization, get to its intended location, and, in particular, arrive on time. Recent research suggests data utilization will improve only when new knowledge is introduced into the proper style of organization life (Pardeck, in press; Pardeck, Murphy, & Callaghan, 1994). Some organizations, for example, encourage departments to compete for information, hide data from one another, and interpret findings in a self-serving manner. In essence, information is simply a weapon in the war of organizational survival. Data will benefit an entire agency, however, only when a reward structure is established that requires persons to share information, collaborate with one another to meet program goals, and promote the overall success of an organization. Some corporations are attempting to facilitate supportive relationships among employees by instituting interdepartmental planning groups, which are charged with developing "key reports." These documents are supposed to detail a data utilization strategy that benefits the whole organization. Furthermore, an organizational structure such as Likert's "linking-pin" can be used to promote group cohesiveness, so that data are understood to constitute public knowledge (Pardeck, Murphy, & Callaghan, 1974). Even the success of "quality circles" depends upon an appropriate definition of knowledge. Organizations need to allow all employees to participate in the planning process.

Computer Systems and Users

Issues must be addressed relative to who will use the computer system. Technicians who computerize the agency are concerned primarily with teaching only those workers who will use the system. The main thrust of this training focuses on the technical knowledge needed to effectively run the computer system. Yet, no effective computer system can be implemented or used effectively on the basis of technical knowledge alone.

Additionally, staff persons must comprehend the purpose of the system, believe they will benefit from its presence, and not find it unduly disruptive to their work schedules. In other words, those who use computers must "buy in" to their worth. This occurs most readily when line employees are able to participate directly in the planning, implementation, and evaluation of an organizational change. Numerous participatory strategies are currently available. Nonetheless, they all seem to provide persons with an important opportunity to experience something new firsthand, in a nonthreatening manner, thereby promoting the development of a positive attitude toward computerization of an agency.

REFERENCES

Boden, M. (1977). *Artificial intelligence and natural man.* New York: Basic Books.

Colby, K. M. (1980). Computer psychotherapists. In J. B. Sidowski, J. W. Johnson, & T. A. Williams (Eds.), *Technology in mental health care delivery systems* (pp. 12-21). Norwood, NJ: Ablex.

Dreyfus, H. & Dreyfus, S. (1986). *Mind over machine.* New York: The Free Press.

Erdman, H. P. & Foster, S. W. (1988). Ethical issues in the use of computer-based assessment. In J. W. Murphy & J. T. Pardeck (Eds.), *Technology and human service delivery* (pp. 71-88). New York: The Haworth Press, Inc.

Karger, H. J. & Kreuger, L.W. (1988). Technology and the not always so human services. In J. W. Murphy & J. T. Pardeck (Eds.), *Technology and human service delivery* (pp. 111-126). New York: The Haworth Press, Inc.

Luhmann, N. (1982). *The differentiation of society.* New York: Columbia University.

Murphy, J. W. & Pardeck, J. T. (1991). *The computerization of human service agencies.* New York: Auburn House.

Pardeck, J. T. (in press). Computer technology in clinical practice: A critical analysis. *Social Work and Social Sciences Review.*

Pardeck, J. T., Murphy, J. W., & Callaghan, K. (1994). Computerization of social services: A critical appraisal. *Scandinavian Journal of Social Welfare, 3 (1),* 2-6.

Schoech, D. (1992). *Human services computing.* New York: The Haworth Press, Inc.

Stuart, R. H. (1988). Social work practice in a high-tech era. In J. W. Murphy & J. T. Pardeck (Eds.), *Technology and human service delivery* (pp. 9-22). New York: The Haworth Press, Inc.

Sociomedical Models and the Epistemology of Risk: The Shortcomings of Medical Decision-Making Research

Dee Vernberg, PhD, MPH

SUMMARY. Sociomedical decision-making models have provided the framework for understanding individual choice regarding health risks and have had an enormous impact on the practice of health education. Recently, some scholars have questioned the usefulness of these models and have called for a new perspective. While some newer decision-making models appear to be unique, it will be shown here that these new approaches remain firmly grounded in value-expectancy tradition.

By examining sociomedical decision-making models with regard to their underlying theory of human action and epistemological assumptions, the similarity of various models will be exposed. The intent of this analysis is to illuminate the inherent limitations of traditional medical decision-making models and to provide a framework for developing a new approach. *[Article copies available for a fee from The Haworth Document Delivery Service: 1-800-342-9678. E-mail address: getinfo@haworth.com]*

Dee Vernberg is Assistant Professor of Communication at the University of Kansas, Lawrence, KS.

Address correspondence to Dee Vernberg, Department of Communication, University of Kansas, Lawrence, KS 66045.

[Haworth co-indexing entry note]: "Sociomedical Models and the Epistemology of Risk: The Shortcomings of Medical Decision-Making Research." Vernberg, Dee. Co-published simultaneously in *Journal of Health & Social Policy* (The Haworth Press, Inc.) Vol. 9, No. 4, 1998, pp. 31-49; and: *Reason and Rationality in Health and Human Services Delivery* (ed: John T. Pardeck, Charles F. Longino, Jr., and John W. Murphy) The Haworth Press, Inc., 1998, pp. 31-49. Single or multiple copies of this article are available for a fee from The Haworth Document Delivery Service [1-800-342-9678, 9:00 a.m. - 5:00 p.m. (EST). E-mail address: getinfo@haworth.com].

31

INTRODUCTION

During the twentieth century, public health demonstrated that a host of infectious diseases could be controlled by employing technical measures that either decreased the communicability of microbes or the susceptibility of people to these agents. Based upon a belief that diseases are caused by natural phenomena that attack the human body, these early prevention approaches tended to minimize the role of individual decision-making in health and disease and instead focused more on physical manipulations to the human body or the environment.

This indifference to the role of human judgment in health and disease changed when the principles underlying the germ theory were found to be inadequate for addressing the emerging public health problems caused by chronic diseases and injuries. Scientists responded to this dilemma by promoting the idea that diseases be studied with multiple causation models. By reconceptualizing disease causation as a product of multiple risk factors, lifestyle emerged as a significant determinant for many of the most prevalent diseases and conditions (Crawford, 1987). Moreover, this rise in the relative importance of the behavioral risk factors redirected the target of prevention from the microbe to individual decision-making.

The notion that people could be influenced through education is not a new strategy in public health, but persuading people to act on the basis of risk arguments has introduced new considerations in health education. For example, instead of promoting a relatively small number of self-protective actions that target microbes (vaccination, personal hygiene, and avoidance of contagious persons), risk factor knowledge results in numerous recommendations that target people's way of life (e.g., exercise, diet, the use of substances such as alcohol, drugs, tobacco; or technologies such as safety belts or smoke alarms). Probabilistic knowledge, however, does not always translate into statements of personal risk. Instead, risk messages summarize the probability of harm for a population or a group. But because risk knowledge is equated with an understanding of cause, recommendations based on this information are viewed as a way to achieve safety or to avoid illness (Slovic, 1987). Medical decision-making research, then, is essentially concerned with how people make decisions under conditions of uncertainty; there have been numerous models developed to examine this phenomenon.

This article will present some of the most common decision-making models that have been used to study health behaviors by addressing the assumptions underlying these approaches. The first part of this investigation will show how the theories of human action advanced by behaviorism, value-expectancy and information processing underlie many key decision-making models. The second part of this inquiry is designed to explain the epistemology of these theories of human action. The goal of this analysis is to reveal the underlying assumptions of how individuals are viewed, the function of reason in behavior and judgment, and the role of the human mind in decision-making. The intent of this discussion is to present a new perspective on decision-making that will illuminate the limitations of traditional medical decision-making research and to provide a foundation for why many scholars are calling for a new conceptualization of decision-making (Centers for Disease Control and Prevention, 1994).

HEALTH BEHAVIOR MODELS

Beginning in the 1950s, medical decision-making studies were undertaken because investigators believed that findings from this research could help them develop effective prevention strategies. The *Health Belief Model,* the *Theory of Reasoned Action,* and *Social Cognitive Theory* will be briefly discussed here because these three models have guided much of the health behavior research, and together these models cover the range of constructs that have been included in other cognitive health behavior models (Zimmerman & Vernberg, 1994). The goal in this discussion is to show how these models have attempted to quantify decision-making. The intent of this section is to show that these approaches are more similar theoretically than they are different, and can be understood as products of behaviorism and value-expectancy theory. Information processing theory also will be introduced since this perspective has been adopted recently by many public health practitioners to conceptualize risk perception and is now being used to develop educational strategies.

The *Health Belief Model* (HBM) has been used more frequently than any other cognitive model to study health-related behavior. Initially developed by the U.S. Public Health Service to study compliance with screening recommendations, the HBM advances the notion that decision-making is influenced by perceptions of risk and expected consequences (positive or negative) of a particular action (Cleary, 1987; Zimmerman & Vernberg, 1994). Human action, then, is viewed as a product of motivation, and the core components of the HBM, for the most part, measure psychological readiness to act. The HBM is comprised of seven components which include perceived susceptibility, perceived severity, perceived benefits and barriers, cues to action, general health motivation, efficacy expectations, and other variables (e.g., demographic variables). Over time, various combinations of these factors have been used to study not only screening behavior, but also lifestyle changes (diet, exercise, etc.), acceptance of immunizations, use of particular therapies, or compliance with medication recommendations (Bertakis, 1986; Brubaker, Prue, & Rychtarik, 1987; Champion, 1985; Janz & Becker, 1984; Kirscht, 1983; Mullen, Hersey, & Iverson, 1987; Rosenstock, 1974; Rosenstock, Strecher, & Becker, 1988).

The *Theory of Reasoned Action* (TRA), sometimes referred to as the *Theory of Planned Behavior* or the *Fishbein-Ajzen Model*, incorporates many of the same ideas as the HBM but the measurement of these percep-tions is approached somewhat differently (e.g., perceived benefits vs. be-lief that a behavior will lead to a certain outcome). The TRA is different from the HBM in three important ways. First, compared to the HBM, the TRA more consistently measures the influence of social factors as defined by *normative expectations and motivations to comply*. Second, the TRA model includes the construct and intention, and it hypothesizes that this variable rather than attitudes or beliefs is the immediate determinant of behavior. Therefore, the function of all other components (beliefs, atti-tudes toward behavior, perceptions of behavioral outcomes or of social norms) is to predict whether or not a person will decide to act. This *a priori* designation of how the different variables in this model are related to each other is the third way that the TRA differs from the HBM. This modeling of variable relationships not only defines how attitudes are re-lated to behavior but specifies how statistical analyses should be con-ducted (Kirscht, 1983; Zimmerman & Vernberg, 1994).

The major contribution that *Social Cognitive Theory* (also previously referred to as Social Learning Theory) has made to the field of medical decision-making is through the introduction of the concept of self-effica-cy. But Social Cognitive Theory (SCT) is also an important model to consider because it provides a theoretical justification for the role of learn-ing in behavior change (Bandura, 1977). What SCT promotes is the idea that behavior is influenced by cognitive expectancies as well as incentives; it also represents an attempt to explain behavior in terms of behavioristic and cognitive learning theories (Kronenfeld & Glik, 1991; Rosenstock, Strecher, & Becker, 1988; Zimmerman & Vernberg, 1994).

Several authors have noted that the constructs included in these three models are quite similar (Mullen, Hersey, & Iverson, 1987; Rosenstock, Strecher, & Becker, 1988; Zimmerman & Vernberg, 1994). Figure 1 shows how these models compare on this dimension.

Figure 1 illustrates that cognition plays a central role in these various models. What may not be so obvious is that these models have adopted a cognitive behaviorist theory of human action. By adhering to this perspec-tive, these models limit the study of cognition by considering only those perceptions that contribute to a rational cost-benefit approach to choice.

FIGURE 1. Comparison of Health Behavior Models

Concept	Models		
	Health Belief Model	Theory of Reasoned Action	Social Cognitive Theory
Risk Perception	Susceptibility Severity	————	Expectancies about environmental cues (beliefs about what leads to what)
Beliefs about self	Self-efficacy	Perceived Behavioral Control	Self-efficacy
Attitudes and Beliefs about health-related action	Benefits Barriers Health motivation	Behavioral expectations Outcome evaluations	Outcome Expectancies
Social Environment (incentives or reinforcements)	Cues to action	Normative expectations Motivations to comply	Modeling Social Support
Mediating or Moderating Variables	Other variables	Intention	Skills

Likewise, culture is restricted to aspects of the human environment (values, norms, knowledge) that relate directly to self-interested action or materially driven intentions (Good, 1985; Sahlins, 1976). While the notion of risk perception is not specifically measured in any of these models and, therefore, not treated as such in the literature, risk perception can be thought about in terms of cause or perceived susceptibility and severity (Kronenfeld & Glik, 1991).

These and other value-expectancy models have had an enormous impact on the study of decision-making; however, a number of scholars have criticized these approaches because specific models, when tested, do not reflect actual decision-making (i.e., the amount of variance in the dependent variable accounted for by the independent variables [R^2] is typically low when these models are tested). In other words, decision-makers often violate the rational principles underlying these models. This finding has led some researchers to question whether people are irrational or whether the decision-making process that people use is unreasonable.

Several alternative models, based on information processing theory, have been proposed to address the deficiencies of the value-expectancy models. One approach, *prospect theory,* advances the idea that people process information differently depending on how a risk choice is framed. For example, behavior change is hypothesized to be more likely if some effort is perceived to virtually eliminate risk as opposed to reducing risk by a certain amount. Therefore, instead of approaching the concept of value as an attribute that can be measured on a scale, prospect theory proposes that value be considered as a change from some reference point (Quattrone & Tversky, 1988). Another finding from prospect theory is that people have predictable biases and inconsistencies when they are asked to think probabilistically (Plous, 1992; Slovic, Fischhoff, & Lichtenstein, 1977).

One of the biases described by prospect theory is referred to as the availability heuristic. This notion states that experience is a major determinant of risk perception. Therefore, people will judge an event to be more likely on the basis of how easy it is to think about, imagine or recall such an event. The availability heuristic also provides an explanation for why publicity is potentially such a powerful intervention or influence on behavior. For example, publicity can either distort perceptions of availability or can correctly inform people so that they can take needed action (Kristiansen, 1983; Plous, 1992; Slovic, Howard, & White, 1982). Because of these and other heuristic findings regarding how people process risk information, many educational messages are now being framed in terms of lifetime risk rather than according to some other shorter metric. In highway safety prevention campaigns, this approach has recently been used. For example, prevention literature may now warn that the "lifetime odds are 1:3 that you will be seriously injured in a traffic crash, and 1 in 100 that you will be killed" (*Drive It Safe,* 1994, p. 1). By framing risk over a 50-year time period (lifetime of auto travel), this theory presumes that people will perceive the risk of being injured or killed in an automobile crash as more likely and will, therefore, take the needed precautions to protect themselves (Slovic, Fischhoff, & Lichtenstein, 1987).

Information processing theory, then, has guided a wide variety of descriptive studies of decision-making, but it has also influenced some newer models that approach preventive behavior initiation and maintenance as a process occurring in stages. These models have also suggested that the effectiveness of interventions may vary depending on which stage of cognitive processing a person is operating (Dreyfus & Dreyfus, 1986; Kronenfeld & Glik; Massaro, 1993; Slovic, Fischhoff, & Lichtenstein, 1977; Weinstein, 1988).

These and other descriptions of how people make decisions suggest that information processing may be the direction that health decision-making research is likely to take in the future. What is conspicuously lacking from the literature on choice behavior or decision-making have been investigations into the epistemological underpinnings of these theories.

DECISION-MAKING THEORY: THEORIES OF HUMAN ACTION AND THE UNDERLYING EPISTEMOLOGY

Behaviorism

Theory of Human Action

Many medical decision-making models have adopted a behavioristic theory of human action. This particular theory of human action advances the idea that behavior is a response to reinforcing factors and can be studied as a stimulus-response functional relationship (Hewitt, 1993; Quill, 1972; Thomson, 1968).

The idea of behavioral reinforcements supports the notion that behavior can be learned and the belief that behavior can change. These ideas are reflected in traditional medical decision-making models as environmental factors (physical and social) that are thought to reinforce behavior. The idea that behavior is driven by future rewards also sustains the central premise of these models: that behavior is goal-oriented (Hewitt, 1993; Thomson, 1968).

Epistemology

Because behaviorism rejects anything considered to be unobservable, such as perceptions or beliefs, thinking or decision-making is not considered to be relevant to human action. In order to sustain this belief, some behaviorists such as J. B. Watson assumed that human consciousness, or the mind, was nonexistent. Other behaviorists such as B. F. Skinner simply treated the human mind as scientifically meaningless, because the presence or absence of subjective factors were considered to be unobservable (Hewitt, 1993; Priest, 1991). In order to consider notions such as cognition, behaviorists approached the human mind as a physical thing. According to Skinner, "all feelings, including fearing and wanting, are bodily, not mental" (Teichman, 1988). Although Skinner was not able to provide any proof for this statement, the idea that "thinking is simply behaving and may be analyzed as such" underlies behavioristic theories (Teichman, 1988).

At the heart of behaviorism is the idea that scientific reason can be used to discover empirical laws that show how a specific response is a function of a particular stimulus. And because reason, measurement and quantification are all important components of scientific method, these natural laws are presumed to be reflected in mathematical relationships. Consequently, the analysis of human behavior is reduced to a correlation between overt stimuli and obvious reactions. This approach assumes that the methods of the natural sciences are appropriate for studying human behavior. Therefore, approaches that incorporate introspective notions are considered to be unscientific (Thomson, 1968; Schwartz, 1978).

By embracing the assumptions of scientific reason, behaviorism promoted a mechanized view of humans as "thing-like" organisms that are controlled by modifying stimuli or reinforcements. By defining humans in material terms, behaviorism accepted a dualistic philosophy of the mind. This position assumes that the body is comprised of two distinct independent entities: the physical and the mental. This segregation of the mental from the physical and the resulting inferiorization of the mind defines humans as mindless entities that simply react to their environment. Like the detached, objective view of the body that René Descartes advanced which suggested that the body would work the same even if no mind were present, the behaviorists promoted the view that human behavior occurs independently of the mind (Chalmers, 1978; Foss & Rothenberg, 1987; Teichman, 1988; The History of Science and Technology, 1988).

Value-Expectancy Models

Theory of Human Action

Cognitive theories, such as value-expectancy, reject the behavioristic position and argue that products of the mind, such as decision-making, are central to understanding behavior (Quill, 1972). In fact, *value-expectancy theory* was developed as an alternative to behaviorism in order to allow subjective factors to be considered in theories of human action. This maneuver was achieved by conceptualizing behavior in terms of an input-output system. By allowing factors such as memory, attention, imagery, and other subjective experiences to be included in the study of human behavior, value-expectancy theory elevated the role of decision-making in human action theories. A major premise of value-expectancy theories is that what a person does bears some relation to his beliefs or expectations regarding the consequences of his behavior. By assuming that behavior is goal oriented rather than simply a reaction to the environment as behaviorism suggests, individuals are viewed as active decision-makers (Feather, 1982; Tyler, 1981).

The value-expectancy model of decision-making is based on the presumption that people will act on the basis of their value of a particular outcome and their perception that a particular action will result in a valued outcome (Maiman & Becker, 1974). This general cost-benefit approach to decision-making reveals the influence of economics in theories of decision-making. For example, like the *expected utility model* developed by the economists John von Neumann and Oskar Morgenstern, value-expectancy models approach decision-making as a rational process of choosing the alternative with the highest utility. Unlike the early economic theories of decision-making, value expectancy incorporates perception in the choice process. The assumption is that people quantify each alternative open to them by weighing the utility of the outcome and multiplying this number by its perceived probability (Plous, 1992; von Neumann, 1947).

The notion of risk perception, then, is an important component in the theory of human action proposed by the value-expectancy models. These perceptions, however, must be rational in order for the cost-benefit calculation to be valid. What this means is that risk perceptions are rational if they mirror objective risk and are uninformed or irrational if they differ. The emphasis on rationality in decision-making is important because reason is thought to be necessary for decisions to be patterned and stable, and for behavior to be understood (Craib, 1984; Good, 1985).

Epistemology

The image of the human mind adopted by the value-expectancy models is a rational mind that acts on the basis of Bayesian statistical principles. Therefore, the purpose of individual decision-making models, such as the HBM, TRA, or SCT, is to explicate how a rational person orders preferences. Because rational choice theories, such as value-expectancy, prescribe the most efficient way to reach a goal, they are sometimes referred to as normative theories. These approaches assume that individuals make decisions that will bring the greatest pleasure or the most predictable results. The role of perception in these models is to reflect accurately estimates of utility which are usually expressed in terms of risk. And the function of the mind is to decide which option is the right one. Value-expectancy theory assumes the rational mind will quantify each of the various options using statistical principles and will choose the alternative with the highest value or probability for success (Craib, 1988; Craib, 1992; Nathanson, 1985).

In value-expectancy theory, the individual is the universal "Economic

Man" who proceeds rationally in pursuit of optimal goals. Inherent in this perspective is a theory of hedonism that defines value as pleasure. Therefore, individuals are reduced to pleasure-seeking entities that only act in order to gain something for themselves. In the realm of health behaviors, the individual is assumed to be avoiding illness or to be seeking health. Whether intentional or not, value-expectancy models presume that individuals act in a somewhat one-dimensional lifeworld by systematically excluding other important considerations (Good, 1985).

Information Processing Theory

Theory of Human Action

Like value-expectancy theory, information processing theory considers decision-making a prerequisite for social action, but information processing suggests that value-expectancy theory is flawed because it promotes the ideal of maximization. Information processing theory advances the notion that people make judgments to reach a satisfactory outcome rather than to obtain the best result. Based on Herbert Simon's theory of *bounded rationality*, humans construct a simplified model of the world and choose the path that satisfies the most important personal needs. What Simon is arguing is that while decisions may not be perfect, as measured by the ideal of maximization, they are adaptive. And decision-making studies should describe this process (Plous, 1992; Simon, 1956; Simon, 1983; Slovic, Kunreuther, & White, 1974).

Information processing theory suggests the idea that people, like computers, respond to information that they receive from the environment. Accordingly, human action is shaped by the way that people process this information. Using the computer as a model, information processing compares human thinking with the problem-solving logic used to program "thinking" in computers. This approach has led to the idea that people use a variety of heuristics in deciding what to do, and that people possess numerous biases that distort their perception (Dreyfus, 1972; Slovic, Fischhoff, & Lichtenstein, 1987; Weizenbaum, 1976; Winograd & Flores, 1986).

Epistemology

Information processing theory uses a computer model to describe how the human mind processes information. Like computers, people are assumed to be symbol-manipulating devices that process information with some type of biological equivalent to a binary on-off switch. Since digital computers essentially count discrete states in order to get results, the human mind is similarly viewed as a device that operates on bits of information according to formal rules. Accordingly, the function of the mind is limited to processing information according to a type of reason that can be expressed as the rules in a computer program. The assumption underlying this view is that the rules the mind uses to make decisions can be formalized, which implies that all knowledge can be expressed in terms of logical binary relations (Dreyfus, 1972; Dreyfus, 1992).

The role of the mind in information processing is central, because, like the computer, it produces information. But, by conceptualizing the brain and mind as computer processors, the mind has been transformed into a mechanical entity. This means that the brain is doing the mechanical computer-like processing that underlies "mental" decision-making. By approaching thinking in terms of a program comprised of *a priori* rules, there is no need for interpretation. Like behaviorism, information processing views human judgment and intuition as irrelevant to human decision-making (Bolter, 1984; Dreyfus & Dreyfus, 1986; Dreyfus, 1992).

With the advent of information processing theory, some scientists began to grapple with ideas regarding the nature of reason. These investigations led to the idea that intelligence could be operationalized and that reason was nothing but a set of rules or heuristics (Bolter, 1984). Beginning with what became known as the Turing Test, and later with the project of artificial intelligence, the logic of computer reason was promoted as the paradigm for what it means to be intelligent or to think. Ultimately, the project of artificial intelligence would support the belief that all human subjective experiences, including insight and intuition, operate according to the rules of reason (Winograd & Flores, 1986; Dreyfus, 1992).

The idea that rational decision-making, like computer reasoning, is a step-wise process of choosing among alternatives is a product of Herbert Simon's concept of bounded rationality. This idea has been influential among decision-making researchers examining self-protective behaviors prior to disasters and is becoming more influential in studies examining other health-related behaviors. The concept of bounded rationality implies that people are inherently deficient because they do not think probabilistically. To compensate, people make decisions using a variety of heuristics in order to reach a satisfactory goal. On the surface, this position may appear to be a new concept of reason, but on closer inspection the maximization principle held by value-expectancy theory is maintained even if it can never be achieved. Therefore, the practical decision-making described by bounded rationality is a rough approximation to this ideal (De Vany, 1996; Winograd & Flores, 1986).

The particular view of the mind and rendition of reason held by information processing serves to reinforce the idea that humans are objects whose behavior can be expressed in precise laws. In fact, by anthropomorphizing the computer as a "thinking machine," humans have been transformed into mechanical information-processors. Accordingly, all subjective thought, including meaning and language, is reduced to the transmission of bits of information that are rule-bound, fixed and independent of the context in which they appear. The assumption is that human experience can be reduced to geometric structures defined by complexly linked matrices. In short, the theory of information processing is the most complete integration of humanity and technology in the history of Western cultures (Bolter, 1984; Winograd & Flores, 1986).

Many of the notions of information processing, such as computer man can solve any task, reflect the optimism of the Enlightenment. But the total mechanization of individuals is antithetical to the spirit of the Enlightenment. The image of individuals as context-free robots or unambivalent pleasure machines ignores and depreciates the consequences of tradition and the deep-seated contextual motives that drive individuals and societies. By defining experience as a game that has well-defined problems that can be solved according to strict rules, culture is ignored and the result is a science that focuses solely on an intellectual world of its own making. The insidious outcome of this approach is that computer rationality has come to define what it is to be human. And when individuals do not act this way, they are viewed as problematic or biased (Bolter, 1984).

Because most medical and public health practitioners do not understand or appreciate the epistemology underlying medical decision-making models, they tend to be somewhat perplexed about why these models have failed to explain behavior. Given the lack of attention that theory receives in most public health settings, many practitioners do not realize that they are adopting findings from studies using information processing theory. In fact, a large part of what professionals now believe about risk perception are really generalizations from studies using the information processing perspective.

As Americans increasingly are expected to take more responsibility for their health, health educators have been searching for ways to foster and encourage this expectation.

Given the epistemological assumptions underlying value-expectancy and information processing theories, it is unlikely that these perspectives will prove useful in this endeavor. This is because these theories model rational learning rather than intelligent behavior. Individuals who operate solely on the model of optimization are not capable actors in the real world because this narrow perspective does not allow them to cope with new situations (De Vany, 1996). The empowerment model of health education is being advanced by some scholars as an alternative to these perspectives.

Empowerment Model

The empowerment model of health education is an approach that attempts to help people assume control over their lives in the context of their social and political environment (Freire, 1973; Rappaport, 1987; Zimmerman & Rappaport, 1988). As a product from the field of adult education, the goal of this approach is to facilitate creative thinking and problem-solving. As such, the empowerment model is not so much concerned with expectations of compliance as it is with creating the conditions for people to make their own informed decisions.

Theory of Human Action

The empowerment model of health education promotes the idea that people are creative actors who make decisions based on interpretations that emerge from the *lifeworld*. What this perspective assumes is that individuals act according to meanings that arise out of language. Unlike the static, rule-bound interpretations that people make in information processing theory, the empowerment model asserts that meanings are variable and can be changed or modified based on experiences (Blumer, 1969; Choi & Murphy, 1992). Human action, then, is bound up and directed toward an experienced world. As Henri Bergson points out, human action is a duration or a "lived through" experience (Giddens, 1993).

Epistemology

The empowerment model perspective is an outgrowth of interpretive philosophies, but can be thought of as adopting some of the epistemological assumptions of phenomenology and postmodernism. In fact, phenomenology and postmodernism make a contribution by showing how experience can be unified without resorting to an idealistic or a materialistic philosophy of the mind. The notion of perception, then, is conceived of in a radically different way.

The empowerment theory attempts to treat the human mind as *intentional*: a term that allows a connection between the mind and the body without eliminating either the mind or physical reality. The notion of intentionality does this by considering human experience and its contents as being intertwined. Therefore, intentional meaning is not abstract but is tied to the world of practical matters (Stewart & Mickunas, 1990; Giddens, 1993; Murphy, 1986).

Perception is also viewed as being intentional, which is to say that "perception is always perception of . . . " This means that perception is more than a reflection of some external reality or a psychological process. Instead, perception is constituted jointly by the perceiver and the perceived. For example, empirical science explains sound as a series of waves that impinge on the ear drum or brain. Phenomenology does not reject this explanation but asserts that this information must be organized by the human mind and is experienced as music, for example. Human experience unifies perception and the object that is perceived, because people do perceive both the subject and the object at the same time. In thinking about the mind and perception as intentional, one can see why subjectivity and objectivity can not and should not be relegated into mutually exclusive categories (Bannan, 1967; Stewart & Mickunas, 1990).

Speech and communication also play an important role in perception because it is through words that an individual's thinking is delivered to him or her. Language, then, is a way that meaning is expressed. Therefore, like perception, language is intentional and expresses intentional activity. Unlike empirical renditions of language that reduce this activity to sounds and visual symbols, phenomenology treats language as "situated" which implies that the meaning of language emerges only within a particular context (Bannan, 1967; Murphy & Choi, 1993; Stewart & Mickunas, 1990). Because the meanings or rules of language are produced by lay actors in the lifeworld and represent knowledge, an understanding of decision-making must consider experiential language (Choi & Murphy, 1992).

By viewing all human activity as intentional, reason can no longer be limited to *a priori* rules that are applied dispassionately regardless of the context. Instead, phenomenologists and postmodernists suggest that researchers approach reason in a "presuppositionless" way. This definition of reason does not reject adopting assumptions or even treating action as being rule-bound. The presuppositionless approach instead rejects the practice of being inattentive to assumptions or simply accepting certain presuppositions as automatically real. By suspending judgment about assumptions, these underlying ideas can be established on a more certain basis. In short, postmodern reason is treated as being contextual (Craib, 1984; Giddens, 1993; Murphy, 1989; Stewart & Mickunas, 1990).

The view of the individual in the empowerment model is more complex than the "economic man" or the robotic homunculi presumed by the value-expectancy or information-processing theory. Instead of defining *a priori* how people should think, the empowerment model seeks to uncover the set of rules that people use to make decisions. For it is only by understanding the interpretive process of intentional beings that socially relevant interventions or policies can be developed.

CONCLUSIONS

As public health practitioners search for strategies that will enhance individuals' capacity to improve their health, attention to the underlying epistemology of strategies is crucial. Otherwise, the public will continue to be viewed as manipulable, causally conditioned, rational utility maximizers or unambivalent pleasure machines, and interventions will remain mechanistic and impersonal (Frazer, 1989). By examining the epistemological assumptions underlying interventions, policy makers may find that many "community oriented" interventions remain firmly grounded in the tradition of behaviorism and fall short of their intended goals. Therefore, notions such as participation, partnership, and collaboration in health care may actually represent empty rhetoric. If practitioners and policy makers truly wish to enhance people's capacity to improve their health, a theory of human action must be embraced that incorporates the notion of *intentionality*.

The empowerment model has great promise if it allows health to be approached as emerging from the lifeworld. By viewing risk as intentional, rather than as an objective measure to be perceived, a more accurate understanding of decision-making may emerge. This knowledge, in turn, has great promise for making health promotion activities more reasonable and more effective.

REFERENCES

American Academy of Orthopaedic Surgeons. (1994). *Drive it safe* [Brochure]. Rosemont, IL: Author.

Bandura, A. (1977). Self-efficacy: Toward a unifying theory of behavioral change. *Psychological Review 84*: 191-215.

Bannan, J. F. (1967). *The philosophy of Merleau-Ponty.* New York: Harcourt, Brace & World, Inc.

Bertakis, K. D. (1986). An application of the health belief model to patient education and compliance: Acute Otitis Media. *Family Medicine 18* (6), 347-350.

Biddle, W. W. (1968). Deflating the community developer. *Community Development Journal 33* (4), 191-194.

Blumer, H. (1969). *Symbolic interactionism: Perspective and method.* Englewood Cliffs: Prentice Hall.

Bolter, J. D. (1984). *Turing's man: Western culture in the computer age.* Chapel Hill: The University of North Carolina Press.

Brubaker, R. G., Prue, D. M., & Rychtarik, R. G. (1987). Determinants of disulfiram acceptance among alcohol patients: A test of the theory of reasoned action. *Addictive Behaviors 12,* 43-51.

Centers for Disease Control and Prevention, Division of Chronic Disease Control and Community Intervention. (1994, September). *Creating capacity: A health education research agenda* (pp. 1-38). Report of a meeting sponsored by the Society for Public Health Education and the Centers for Disease Control and Prevention. Atlanta, GA: Centers for Disease Control.

Chalmers, A. F. (1978). *What is this thing called science? An assessment of the nature and status of science and its methods.* St. Lucia: University of Queensland Press.

Champion, V. L. (1985). Use of the health belief model in determining frequency of breast self-examination. *Research in Nursing & Health 8,* 373-379.

Choi, J. M., & Murphy, J. W. (1992). *The politics and philosophy of political correctness.* Westport: Praeger.

Cleary, P. (1987). Why people take precautions against health risks. In N. D. Weinstein (Ed.), *Taking care: Understanding and encouraging self-protective behavior* (pp. 119-149). Cambridge: Cambridge University Press.

Craib, I. (1984). *Modern social theory: From Parsons to Habermas.* Great Britain: Wheatsheaf Books.

Craib, I. (1992). *Modern social theory: From Parsons to Habermas.* New York: St. Martin's Press.

Crawford, R. (1987). Cultural influences on prevention and the emergence of a new health consciousness. In N. D. Weinstein (Ed.), *Taking care: Understanding and encouraging self-protective behavior* (pp. 95-113). Cambridge: Cambridge University Press.

De Vany, A. (1996). Putting a human face on rational expectations: A book review. *Journal of Economic Dynamics and Control 20,* 811-817.

Dreyfus, H. L. (1972). *What computers can't do: A critique of artificial reason.* New York: Harper & Row Publishers.

Dreyfus, H. L. (1992). *What computers still can't do.* Cambridge and London: The MIT Press.

Dreyfus, H. L., & Dreyfus, S. E. (1986). *Mind over machine: The power of human intuition and expertise in the era of the computer.* New York: The Free Press.

Feather, N. T. (1982). Introduction and overview. In N. T. Feather (Ed.), *Expectations and actions: Expectancy-value models in psychology* (pp. 1-4). Hillsdale: Lawrence Erlbaum Associates.

Foss, L., & Rothenberg, K. (1987). *The second medical revolution: From biomedicine to infomedicine.* Shambhala: New Science Library.

Fraser, N. (1989). *Unruly practices: Power, discourse, and gender in contemporary social theory.* Minneapolis: University of Minnesota Press.

Freire, P. (1973). *Education for critical consciousness.* New York: Seabury Press.

Giddens, A. (1993). *New rules of sociological method: A positive critique of interpretive sociologies* (2nd ed.). Stanford, CA: Stanford University Press.

Good, B. (1985). Explanatory models and care seeking: A critical account. In S. McHugh & T. M. Vallis (Eds.), *Illness behavior: A multidisciplinary model.* New York: Plenum Press.

Hewitt, J. P. (1993). *Self and society: A symbolic interactionist social psychology* (6th ed.). Boston: Allyn and Bacon.

The history of science and technology: A narrative chronology. (1988). In Facts on File, Inc. Prehistory-1900. New York: Facts on File.

Janz, N. K., & Becker, M. (1984). The health belief model: A decade later. *Health Education Quarterly 11* (1), 1-47.

Kirscht, J. P. (1983). Preventive health behavior: A review of research and issues. *Health Psychology 2* (3), 277-301.

Kristiansen, C. M. (1983). Newspaper coverage of diseases and actual mortality statistics. *European Journal of Social Psychology 13,* 193-194.

Kronenfeld, J. J., & Glik, D. C. (1991). Perceptions of risk: Its applicability in medical sociological research. *Research in the Sociology of Health Care 9,* 307-334.

Maiman, L. A., & Becker, M. H. (1974). The health belief model: Origins and correlates in psychological theory. *Health Education Monographs 2* (4), 336-353.

Massaro, D. W. (1993). Information processing models: Microscopes of the mind. *Annual Review of Psychology 44,* 383-425.

Mullen, P. D., Hersey, J. C., & Iverson, D. C. (1987). Health behavior models compared. *Social Science and Medicine 24* (11), 973-981.

Murphy, J. W. (1986). Phenomenological social science: Research in the public interest. *The Social Science Journal 23* (3), 327-343.

Murphy, J. W. (1989). *Postmodern social analysis and criticism.* New York: Greenwood Press.

Murphy, J. W., & Choi, J. M. (1993). Decentering social relations. In J. W. Murphy & D. L. Peck (Eds.), *Open institutions* (pp. 161-176). Westport: Praeger.

Nathanson, S. (1985). *The ideal of rationality.* Atlantic Highlands, NJ: Humanities Press International, Inc.

Plous, S. (1992). *The psychology of judgment and decision making.* Philadelphia, PA: Temple University Press.

Priest, S. (1991). *Theories of the mind.* Boston: Houghton Mifflin Company.

Quattrone, G. A., & Amos, T. (1988). Contrasting rational and psychological analyses of political choice. *American Political Science Review 82,* 719-736.

Quill, W. G. (1972). *Subjective psychology: A concept of mind for the behavioral sciences and philosophy.* New York: Spartan Books.

Rappaport, J. (1987). Terms of empowerment/examples of prevention: Towards a theory for community psychology. *American Journal of Communication Psychology 15* (2), 121-148.

Rosenstock, I. M. (1974). Historical origins of the health belief model. *Health Education Monographs 2* (4), 328-335.

Rosenstock, I. M., Strecher, V. J., & Becker, M. H. (1988). Social learning theory and the health belief model. *Health Education Quarterly 15* (2), 175-183.

Sahlins, M. (1976). *Culture and practical reason.* Chicago: The University of Chicago Press.

Schwartz, B. (1978). *Psychology of learning behavior.* New York: W. W. Norton and Company, Inc.

Simon, H. A. (1956). Rational choice and the structure of the environment. *Psychological Review 63,* 129-138.

Simon, H. A. (1983). *Reason in human affairs.* Stanford, CA: Stanford University Press.

Slovic, P. (1987). Perception of risk. *Science 236,* 280-285.

Slovic, P., Fischhoff, B., & Lichtenstein, S. (1982). Facts versus fears: Understanding perceived risk. In D. Kahneman, P. Slovic, & A. Tversky (Eds.), *Judgment under uncertainty: Heuristics and biases.* Cambridge, MA: Cambridge University Press.

Slovic, P., Fischhoff, B., & Lichtenstein, S. (1977). Behavioral decision theory. *Annual Review of Psychology 28* (3), 1-39.

Slovic, P., Fischhoff, B., & Lichtenstein, S. (1987). Behavioral decision theory perspectives on protective behavior. In N. D. Weinstein (Ed.), *Taking care: Understanding and encouraging self-protective behavior* (pp. 14-41). Cambridge: Cambridge University Press.

Slovic, P., Howard, K., & White, G. (1974). Decision processes, rationality, and adjustment to natural hazards. In G. F. White (Ed.), *Natural hazards: Local, national, global* (pp. 187-205). New York: Oxford University Press.

Stewart, D., & Mickunas, A. (1990). *Exploring phenomenology: A guide to the field and its literature.* Athens: Ohio University Press.

Teichman, J. (1988). *Philosophy and the mind.* Oxford: Basil Blackwell.

Thomson, R. (1968). *The pelican history of psychology.* Middlesex: Penguin Books.

Tyler, L. E. (1981). More stately mansions–psychology extends its boundaries. *Annual Review of Psychology 32,* 1-20.

von Neumann, J., & Morgenstern, O. (1947). *Theory of games and economic behavior.* Princeton: Princeton University Press.

Weinstein, N. D. (1988). The precaution adoption process. *Health Psychology 7* (4), 355-386.

Weizenbaum, J. (1976). *Computer power and human reason: From judgment to calculation.* San Francisco: W. H. Freeman and Company.

Winograd, T., & Flores, F. (1986). *Understanding computers and cognition: A new foundation for design.* Norwood: Ablex Publishing Corporation.

Zimmerman, M., & Rappaport, J. (1988). Citizen participation, perceived control and psychological empowerment. *American Journal of Communication Psychology, 16*(5), 725-750.

Zimmerman, R. S., & Vernberg, D. (1994). Models of preventive health behavior: Comparison, critique, and meta-analysis. *Advances in Medical Sociology 4*, 45-67.

Community-Based Epidemiology: Community Involvement in Defining Social Risk

Mark H. Smith, PhD

SUMMARY. In traditional epidemiologic research, the concept of risk emerges from a biomedical paradigm which draws heavily upon Cartesian-Newtonian ontological assumptions. Rational assessment of individual risk is based on a culturally conditioned metatheoretical framework that seeks specific causes for specific disease conditions. This leads to the identification of "risk factors" that can be individually modified. Research within this orientation tends to produce interpretations of data which further condition and mold cultural understanding of individual and social risks and the available choices that can be made to modify these risks. Community-based eco-epidemiology balances reductionist tendencies of individual risk-factor analysis against social context and local knowledge gained through community involvement in the research process. The community-based partnership model can contribute to a greater understanding of the interrelatedness of social problems and individual risks on the part of community participants and researchers alike. *[Article copies available for a fee from The Haworth Document Delivery Service: 1-800-342-9678. E-mail address: getinfo@haworth.com]*

Mark H. Smith is Research Assistant Professor and Associate Director of the Center for Community Research in the Section on Social Sciences and Health Policy, Department of Public Health Sciences, Bowman Gray School of Medicine, Winston-Salem, NC 27157.

[Haworth co-indexing entry note]: "Community-Based Epidemiology: Community Involvement in Defining Social Risk." Smith, Mark H. Co-published simultaneously in *Journal of Health & Social Policy* (The Haworth Press, Inc.) Vol. 9, No. 4, 1998, pp. 51-65; and: *Reason and Rationality in Health and Human Services Delivery* (ed: John T. Pardeck, Charles F. Longino, Jr., and John W. Murphy) The Haworth Press, Inc., 1998, pp. 51-65. Single or multiple copies of this article are available for a fee from The Haworth Document Delivery Service [1-800-342-9678, 9:00 a.m. - 5:00 p.m. (EST). E-mail address: getinfo@haworth.com].

INTRODUCTION

Risk assessment is among the central activities of epidemiology, which is the study of the distribution and determinants of disease. The concept of "risk" is integral to the language of epidemiology, a language that includes the "risk-ratio," or "relative risk," and the "population attributable risk." The ability of epidemiology to quantify health risks has propelled the field to a position of public and scientific respect. Among the many successes of epidemiologic risk factor identification are included the discovery that cholera was a result of contamination of well water with sewage and that pellagra was due to a nutritional deficiency; the demonstration of the association between cigarette smoking and lung cancer; and the discovery of the relationship between sex hormones and endometrial cancer. Past accomplishments in identifying and quantifying health risks have led to rising expectations—on the part of the media, policy makers and the general public—of ongoing discoveries, even as epidemiologists increasingly confront the possibility that epidemiology is "facing its limits" (Taubes, 1995).

At the Pan American Epidemiology Congress in 1995, keynote speaker Columbia University epidemiologist Mervyn Susser suggested that epidemiology is on the verge of "a new era" (*Epidemiology Monitor*, 1995). Susser and Susser (1996, I) describe three eras in the development of epidemiology. The first era, that of sanitary statistics in the early 19th century, was accompanied by public health preventive measures such as sewage treatment and sanitary improvements. The second era of infectious disease epidemiology, lasting from the late nineteenth century through the first half of the twentieth century, was driven by the theory of specific etiology and led to procedures to interrupt transmission of, or otherwise combat, specific microbes. The current era, or epoch, is that of chronic disease epidemiology, and is characterized by biostatistical analysis of data on exposures and disease status. These exposures can be to drugs, foods, environmental contaminants, social conditions, or relationships. Models are tested to determine whether these exposures constitute health risks and should be considered as risk factors. The general theme of epidemiologic research in this current epoch is to isolate specific independent risk factors through controls designed to remove the effects of other factors and to assign a magnitude to these risks to health. The preventive approach, favored in this evolutionary era, is designed to control the risk factors by modifying health behaviors or environmental factors. The emerging paradigm described by Susser is one in which epidemiology begins to think more broadly about health and disease, and looks beyond individual risk factors to consider the social, cultural, economic, and political context in which health and disease occur. This context may be the local community, national and international economic and political structures and processes.

The overarching questions addressed by this paper are these: If the new era in epidemiologic risk assessment entails going beyond isolating risk factors to develop an understanding of the relationship between individual behaviors and broader social and environmental contexts, can community involvement in defining risk contribute to the emergent paradigm in epidemiological research? And what are the implications of community-based epidemiology for our understanding of risk and rationality?

The Limits of Epidemiology

Almost daily, the results of health studies in epidemiological research, designed to assess the risks of foods, drugs, pesticides, other environmental toxins, and a variety of personal and social behaviors are reported. These reports result in economic, social and political reactions, whether it is updated New Year's resolutions, increased sales of vitamins, low-fat cookbooks, self-help books, origin of support groups, and the spawning of legislative and regulatory actions.

Epidemiologic assessment of individual health risk plays an important role in the development of individual and social perceptions of health risk, has led to many public health benefits, but has also created what Lewis Thomas referred to as an "epidemic of anxiety" (Taubes, 1995, p. 164). The social reality that emerges from epidemiologic research, as interpreted by communications media, is one in which each food, beverage, drug, occupation, social status, residential location, and behavior pattern is assigned a risk, where everything is "more" or "less" risky in terms of health and well-being, and the path to health is through strategies that avoid these risks. The public is subjected to an onslaught of often contradictory reports regarding the dangers of all manner of risk factors, from power line electromagnetic fields and brain cancer, to hair dyes and lymphomas, to coffee and pancreatic cancer. Unfortunately, the public, and typically the media, do not have the knowledge of research methodology to interpret the validity and significance of new stories about health risks (Mann, 1995).

Despite the public confusion and anxiety over inconsistent epidemiologic reports, it is common to consider epidemiologic methods as the "gold standard" because these methods allow us to assess human health risk directly (Wartenberg & Simon, 1995). By measuring exposures and potentially confounding associated characteristics of individuals, over a period of time, epidemiologic methods provide a powerful means of isolating the effects of clinically significant risk factors. The history of epidemiology is the story of development of ever more powerful and refined methods of assessing health risk: the cross-sectional field survey, case-control studies, prospective cohort studies, multivariate statistical analysis, and the ultimate in modern research methodology–the randomized clinical trial. The randomized double-blinded controlled clinical trial is the most powerful method known to science for isolating and quantifying the effect of a drug, food, or behavioral risk factor, net the effect of other factors.

These epidemiological and biostatistical methods, impressive as they are, are not without their limitations. When it comes to addressing complex conditions, chronic diseases such as heart disease and cancer, and the degenerative conditions associated with aging, isolating risk factors is less successful at explanation and intervention. Some people who have none of the known risk factors for heart disease succumb to the disease, while others who have multiple risk factors survive to old age. Participants at the Pan American Epidemiology Conference described a number of shortcomings of the individual risk factor approach (Koopman, 1995):

1. It has difficulty integrating molecular risk factors with behavioral and social risk factors.

Epidemiology could be characterized as a well-developed epistemology with an underdeveloped ontology. Epidemiologists have at their disposal a bulging toolbox filled with an array of methodological and statistical techniques to answer questions about the distribution and determinants of health and disease. The discipline is generally atheoretical, operating on the basis of what Susser calls the "black box paradigm," described as "connecting exposure with outcome based on the probability of the relationship without the necessity of explaining the connecting links" (Koopman, 1995, p. 7). As a general principle, epistemology (how we know what we think we know) serves to inform ontology (what we think we know). The epistemology of risk-factor epidemiology tends to correspond to the ontological foundations of the biomedical paradigm of health and disease. This paradigm has been described and critiqued extensively elsewhere, but may be briefly characterized as acceptance of the theory of specific etiology (one disease, one cause), the Cartesian split between mind and body, and the reduction of disease etiology to biophysiological mechanisms (Longino & Murphy, 1995; Foss, 1994; Dossey, 1982).

From its early roots in the field research which led to a discovery that a London cholera epidemic had been caused by contaminated drinking water, epidemiology has had a strong tradition of population-based research and a concern for the relationship between the health of individuals and the communities in which they live. The public health orientation of epidemiology contributed to improvements in human health through regulation and improvements in sanitation, clean water supplies, and sewage treatment. The success of the germ theory and the development of biostatistical methods favored the eventual eclipse of the public health emphasis, however. This can be seen, to some extent, with the status of population statistics within the field of epidemiology. Population statistics were once highly valued as a window upon the social context of disease. Now, such aggregated data, usually referred to as "ecologic" data, tend to be denigrated as second rate data compared to individual-level data. This is caused by concern about the ecological fallacy: that of applying aggregate data to assessing individual risk. When we compare exposures and disease patterns in aggregated populations, we do not know whether those who have been exposed are those who contract the disease. This concern over the possibility of committing the ecologic fallacy has led to a marked aversion to population statistics and a tendency to emphasize bio-behavioral individual factors to the neglect of contextual understanding. Hence, despite the fact that social ecology and environmental factors are not at all unfamiliar to epidemiology, the field lacks the metatheoretical foundation to construct explanations that incorporate molecular risk factors with measurements of social and behavioral characteristics.

2. It cannot identify risk factors which are not identifiable in terms of their action upon individuals at risk or whose origin lies in the interaction between individuals or in social or political organization.

Epidemiology, like other disciplines using quantitative measurements, tends to operate similarly to the person who looks for his lost keys under the streetlight because that's where the light is better. Epidemiologists tend to measure those things that are relatively easy to measure. Cultural, economic, social, and political factors possibly related to the situation of interest are typically not measured, either because these risk factors are difficult to measure, or because these factors are not compatible with the underlying assumptions. Proponents of "new-paradigm" medicine, like Dossey (1991) and Chopra (1993), suggest that the meaning that events have for people makes a big difference in the impact these events have on their disease or health risk. Meaning, though, is not supposed to make a difference from a biomedical perspective, and is difficult to measure in any case, so meaning is not measured or considered in the analysis. Evidence is mounting that not only absolute levels of poverty but also the relative spread of incomes impact health and morbidity (Marmot, Bobak, & Smith, 1995; Wilkinson, 1992), but inequitable distribution of the gross national product is rarely examined in epidemiology because these issues are considered "too political." Epidemiologists control for the effects of socioeconomic status; public health and social services are left to mitigate these effects, and thus social allopathy mirrors medical allopathy.

3. It cannot predict accurately the absolute or relative effects of alternative interventions because its quantitative models do not conform to the behavior of the causal systems in which the interventions are to be executed.

This point is illustrated by the debate centered around the Office of Alternative and Complementary Medicine (OACM). The OACM, an office of the National Institutes of Health, is charged with assessing the effectiveness of a wide range of so-called "alternative" therapies for various health conditions. These alternative interventions may include acupuncture, yoga, meditation, prayer, herbal treatments, or holistic lifestyle modification. One side in this debate demands that these alternative therapies be evaluated with the same methods used to evaluate new drugs and clinical procedures: randomized prospective cohort studies and randomized clinical trials. The other side of the debate argues that an epistemology designed to isolate specific effects by controlling out confounders is inadequate to assess interventions based on different ontological grounds.

Dean Ornish demonstrated that, through the combined practice of implementing a low-fat diet, yoga exercises, and meditation, heart disease could be halted and even reversed without drugs (Ornish, 1992). His work was criticized on the grounds that the study design did not allow the components of the intervention to be isolated; there was no way to know how much impact each component contributed to the observed effect. His response was that detractors had missed the point: these parts cannot be isolated and separated; they are integral parts of the whole. From this ontological perspective, risk factors are not isolated, but are integral parts of the whole situation that includes many dimensions operating simultaneously: biophysical, psychological, social, economic, political, cultural, environmental, and spiritual.

During the last twenty years, epidemiological research has made important strides in including sociodemographic, psychosocial and quality of life measures in studies, though the tendency is to regard these as control variables rather than as important theoretical components of the causal web. In manner analogous to the way language constrains thought, methodology constrains research. The stock-in-trade for much epidemiology is the risk-ratio–the probability of experiencing the condition in question with a factor present relative to the probability without that factor. In order to use the multivariate statistical procedures such as logistic regression that produce estimates of relative risk, the researcher is habituated to choose as dependent variables disease conditions and to search for independent risk factors, rather than to examine the synergistic complex of factors that work together to produce health.

4. It tends to make epidemiologists focus on individuals in their search for causes and to ignore social and political factors such as organizational structure or the generation and use of political power not associated with individuals.

If, as has been suggested, the dominant paradigm in epidemiological and biomedical research is based on Newtonian-Cartesian physics, the emergent paradigm is based on a quantum-relativistic ontology, an understanding of a universe in which nothing exists as a thing by itself, but only has existence in relation to everything else. This view denies the classical mechanistic view of the analyzability of the world into separately existing parts (Bohm, 1982).

The difference in these two paradigmatic perspectives has a parallel in the two great branches of Buddhism: Mahayana, the Great Raft, and Hinayana, the Little Raft. The Little Raft school believes that the emancipation of the individual is not contingent on the salvation of others. The Great Raft school holds that the spiritual destiny and fate of the individual is linked to the fate of all. The Great Raft view is exemplified by the definition of health held by the World Health Organization as a state of complete social, psychological, and physical well-being: no one can be fully healthy and whole until everyone is healthy. This orientation is gaining support from research at the University of North Carolina which suggests that viruses attacking malnourished individuals may mutate dangerously to enable the virus to sicken healthy individuals who would normally not be susceptible, leading one researcher to comment, "We are our brother's keeper, because we are affected by what happens" (Associated Press, 1966).

Susser calls the emerging era in epidemiology "ecologism," or "eco-epidemiology." This perspective sees the individual as embedded in a seamless web of relationships, including cultural systems, social, economic, and political systems at the local, national, and international levels. Instead of studying the individual reduction in risk from heart disease resulting from a reduction in dietary saturated fat, an ecologic approach might examine the individual and social risk resulting from the cultural, economic, and political support for a high-fat, meat-based diet. In addition, such an analysis would consider the ancillary risks such as environmental contamination from concentrated animal wastes, the relationship between antibiotic-resistant bacteria and feeding antibiotics to livestock, and the destruction of tropical rainforests to satisfy demand for beef.

COMMUNITY-BASED RESEARCH

With epidemiology ostensibly poised for transition to a new epoch of ecological-oriented research, community-based research approaches gain greater salience. Community-based research differs from traditional population-based epidemiology by virtue of greater involvement of the community in the research process in roles that are usually reserved for the research team and project sponsors. Modern community-based research is heir to several disparate community organization and development traditions. For the purposes of this paper, the relevant antecedents are traced to those overlapping bodies of literature regarding Third World development and rural community development research.

In the post-World War II era, massive national worldwide development programs were undertaken to raise living standards and raise incomes. These programs, financed by the International Monetary Fund and the World Bank, were typically grand, expensive public-works such as hydroelectric dams, highways, and airports. With certain notable exceptions, such as some Pacific Rim nations, these development plans did not work out as planned. Instead of healthy countries and communities, the outcome in many cases was massive indebtedness, increases in wealth inequality, social and cultural turmoil, poverty, and violence. Eventually, some development planners began to question their assumptions. In a classic 1976 article, Everett Rogers described what he called the "passing of the dominant paradigm" (Rogers, 1976, p. 121). A number of important parallels can be observed between this shift in community development paradigms and the shift in thinking in epidemiological and biomedical research. Main elements of the dominant development paradigm are:

1. *Economic growth*: The principle measures of development were per capita income and gross national product; if these measures were rising, it was assumed that everything else would take care of itself.
2. *Capital-intensive technology*: pour money, technicians, experts, and technology into solving the problem.
3. *Centralized planning:* This was top-down development, guided by university and think-tank experts.
4. *Primarily internal causes of underdevelopment*: If countries did not develop as expected, the fault was in their "traditional" practices and beliefs, and not those of modern Western, developed nations.

According to Rogers, the alternative to the dominant paradigm could be characterized by an emphasis on equality of distribution (the trickle-down theory was not working). Rather than capital-intensive technology, emphasis was placed on quality of life and integration of traditional and modern systems in a country, as well as greater emphasis being placed on intermediate-level and labor-intensive technology. Rather than central planning, the alternative approach involves an emphasis on self-reliance in development and popular participation in decentralized self-development planning and execution. The alternative to internal causes of underdevelopment, as a redefinition of the problem, is an understanding of internal and external causes of underdevelopment (such as might be rooted in inequities and distortions in the international economic and political systems).

This call for a paradigm shift was directed to international development planners, but was heard by rural community development planners and rural sociologists in the United States, who realized that the shortcomings of the dominant development paradigm were evident in rural development efforts in this country. Considerable attention was accorded the need for popular participation in decentralized self-development planning and execution. Community analysis, community leadership development, and the community partnership model have become commonplace in Cooperative Extension programs and land-grant university rural development research. What makes this research community-based, and not just research in a community, is the involvement of the community in defining the scope of the research, setting priorities, helping to develop research questions, and contributing to the process of interpreting the meaning of the data.

The parallels between Roger's call for a new development paradigm relative to the proposed shift in epidemiologic research paradigms are readily apparent. The new paradigm of ecologism calls for a de-emphasis on high-tech curative medicine and more emphasis on a holistic understanding of disease causation and prevention; a shift from top-down research initiatives run by university experts and conducted on passive communities of respondents to a greater involvement of communities in each phase of the research process; and the shift from health, as the result of mainly internal forces, to a broader understanding of internal and external systems (ecologism).

How does this collaboration between the research team and the community contribute to the new era in ecological epidemiology and a corresponding new approach to the social construction of risk? What are the potential benefits of this approach, and what are the limitations? In addressing these issues, a number of vital issues converge around what can be called the measurement problem. This problem has its roots in the discoveries of Einstein and the great quantum physicists, Heisenberg, Bohr, and Schroedinger. Under the physics of Newton and Descartes, there was unquestionably a solid objective universe that could be understood by the subjective mind by analyzing the parts of the whole. This view assumed that reality is objective, deterministic, and predictable. Newtonian physics worked very well in many spheres, such as space flight. The quantum physicists discovered, however, that at the sub-atomic level, the universe is not solid at all, but is made up of probability waves, vibrations and frequencies, existing in a state of potentiality rather than actuality. They discovered that if they measured the location of an electron, that they could not measure its velocity; and, if they measured the velocity, they could not measure the location with any certainty. Heisenberg referred to this as the principle of indeterminacy (a term he preferred to the Uncertainty Principle): the state of the electron is indeterminant, having a certain probability of existing in a certain state. The physicists discovered that depending on the method of measurement, electrons would reveal themselves as either particles or waves. The state of the physical entity was determined by the act of measurement itself. Using the most rational of experimental methodology, they discovered that, despite the thick glass separating them from the experimental apparatus, they were not objectively measuring an objective reality. They were subjectively involved in bringing about the reality they observed. Ontological assumptions that emerge from these discoveries are intersubjectivity, probability, indeterminism, and nonlocal causality (Overman, 1989).

Even though the ontological foundation of modern science has undergone revolutionary change, the epistemology of science is slow to change. The ideal in the philosophy and practice of science remains that of the objective observer and analyst taking objective measurements of an objective reality. In the social sciences, the discovery of the "Hawthorne Effect" confirms the applicability of the indeterminacy principle that every measuring process has a reactive element as applied to society. The Hawthorne Effect refers to a study of the impact of various workplace environmental changes on productivity, wherein the researchers found that productivity increased regardless of the environmental modification; it was the act of being studied that made the difference.

Consider, if you will, the act of distributing a questionnaire or administering a telephone survey to assess health risk and health need. The respondent is asked to rate overall health as excellent, very good, good, fair, or poor. He may never have thought of his health in these terms before, but the respondent selects a measurement among categories decided by the observer. To ask how much impact that measurement of self-rated health has on the subsequent health of the individual subject of the measurement is not a frivolous question. We know that self-reported health is the single best predictor of subsequent morbidity and mortality, surpassing clinical diagnosis (Kaplan, Barell, & Lusky, 1988). Why self-rated health is such a powerful predictor of subsequent health is not known with any certainty. In part, it may be that the individual has direct knowledge through awareness of symptoms and signs of disease of his health status. Quantum theory raises another possibility, however, that the act of measurement itself–asking and answering the question, "How would you rate your overall health?" may be reactive with the respondent's health.

The community-based researcher walks around that glass wall that separates the researcher from the sampling frame, from the pool of participants, from society out there, and walks into what Vernberg and Murphy describe as the life-world, where there is a "collapse of dualism" and where "reason is contextual" (1996, p. 131). So now, instead of an objective observer taking measurements, the researcher is a part of a community that includes institutions and individuals that take measurements and study various parts of itself.

Since the researcher is a subjective participant in the community partnership, there is now no illusory possibility that the research process will be non-reactive with the system studied. In the social ecology of the community partnership, the researcher is in the role of the expert, so the opportunity to influence the reactivity of the research is magnified. Since one of the main reasons for involving the community is to avoid imposing the researcher's models, constructs and agendas on the assessment of community health and risk, methods are employed to de-emphasize the role of the researcher, and emphasize the importance of all the various points of view expressed in the community partnership. Recruitment of partnership members is aimed at finding articulate spokespersons for the widest range of relevant perspectives, interests, constituencies.

Through a process of mutual education and discussion, the partnership determines the scope of the assessment and sets the priorities for the research questions. This process is consistent with the requirement of the new development paradigm for local popular participation in decentralized self-development planning and execution. It also tends to counter the tendency to emphasize individual risk factors by returning focus to the community. Reductionist tendencies are countered by the breadth of perspectives on the sources of health risks. Where one locates social risk in a lack of primary care physicians, another sees a lack of public health education and wellness promotion; someone else will point to the effects of poverty, poor living conditions, and lack of access to care; others may draw attention to cultural factors, crises in families, and lack of psychosocial supports.

All of these various partial points of view do not necessarily constitute an ecological analysis or complete understanding of individual and social health risk. They can contribute to an appreciation of the complexity of the factors intertwined with health and risk, and can help ensure that the research assessment process does not neglect to consider questions of relevance to the intersubjective meaning system of the community.

The community-based process is compatible with the tenets of new-epoch epidemiology, but the methodological tools available to epidemiologists have not yet adapted. Because no single methodology is adequate to the task of assessing health needs, community-based risk or needs assessment often use convergent analysis, triangulation, or other multiple method techniques (Campbell & Fiske, 1959). In convergent analysis, secondary data populations statistics are juxtaposed and overlaid with traditional mail or telephone surveys, which are then overlaid with information obtained from focus groups. Attention is given to those areas where these multiple methods overlap and converge. These streams of data are fed back to the community partnerships, which assist in interpreting the meaning of the data. The aim of this approach is not so much to obtain an objective assessment or estimation of social health risk, but to promote a convergence of perspectives around an intersubjective understanding of health needs and risks.

In principle, with each step in the assessment process, community involvement will produce a broader, more authentic assessment and will increase community buy-in to the process. This will make it more likely that the assessment action recommendations will be acted on through subsequent follow-through interventions. There are, however, certain limitations to community-based research. The community-based partnership model moves towards an ecological understanding inasmuch as it tends to emphasize the individual as embedded in a rich context of relationships, employment, church and other activities. There is a danger, however, that the previously observed limitation inherent in the individual risk-factor approach will be repeated at the local community level, with the community viewed in isolation from the social, political, economic, and cultural systems in which it is embedded. Many problems, needs, and risks faced by individuals in communities are rooted in state and national political policies and regulations, national and international economic policies, and broad cultural and social trends and forces. Many of these risks and problems are very difficult to address effectively at the local community level, whether this is a neighborhood, a town, or a county.

One of those locally intractable problems is that of inequality–recall that Rogers' first principle of his new paradigm of development was equality of distribution. That inequality may be reflected in the composition of the partnership. The partnership model is very similar in essence to the democratic pluralistic model of political power. The pluralistic model views politics as a process of competition and accommodation among many different interest groups and factions, which balance and check each other, so that out of this process comes policies roughly representing the public interest. Community power studies have provided considerable reason to suspect that systemic inequalities on economic levels will carry over into public policy levels. Efforts should be made to recruit partners who will act as spokespersons for the needy and disadvantaged, the working poor, racial minorities, on an equal status basis. However, everyone will know that some persons and interests are more equal than others. Patterns of deference based on socioeconomic inequality may combine with patterns of deference based on expertise and authority. Special care must be taken to minimize the tendency for the views of the research team, physicians, and government authorities to carry greater weight in the process of interpreting the data and developing recommendations and action steps.

CONCLUSIONS

The proponents of a "new epoch" in epidemiology contend that the value of the shift to eco-epidemiology lies in public health improvements. The means for accomplishing these improvements entails balancing the reductionist search for universal causal laws with a recognition of the complexity and multidimensionality of human life (Susser & Susser, 1996, II) to "emphasize the importance of diversity and local knowledge rather than only searching for universal relationships" (Pearce, 1996). Obtaining that diversity and local knowledge can be facilitated through community-based assessment of needs and social risks.

The community development process used in community-based research contributes to a recognition of health itself as a measure of community development. The community partnership model typical of community-based research encourages a shift away from overemphasis on individual risk factors and an acknowledgment of social risks. Gradually, communities may develop an appreciation of the risks of radical social inequality; the risks of neglecting health education; the social risks of sending mixed messages about sex and responsibility; the risks of cultural promotion of animal versus plant-based diets; the risks of over-reliance on market solutions to health care problems. Involvement of the community in the construction and understanding of health risks points us away from the small raft philosophy of health toward the philosophy of the Great Raft.

REFERENCES

Bohm, D. (1982). *Wholeness and the implicate order.* Boston: Routledge.
Campbell, D.T. & Fiske, D.W. (1959). Convergent and discriminant validation by the multi-tract multi-method matrix. *Psychological Bulletin, 56,* 81-105.
Chopra, D. (1993). *Ageless body, timeless mind.* New York: Harmony Books.
Dossey, L. (1982). *Space, time, and medicine.* Boulder: Shambhala.
Dossey, L. (1991). *Meaning and medicine.* New York: Bantam Books.
Epidemiology Monitor. (1995). Susser discusses "ecologism" as new paradigm. *Epidemiology Monitor, 16,* 6:1,7.
Foss, L. (1994). Medical ontology: Is it time for a new medical discipline? *Advances, 10, 4:* 67-70.
Kaplan, G., Barell, V., & Lusky, A. (1988). Subjective state of health and survival in elderly adults. *Journal of Gerontology, 43, 4:* S114-120.
Koopman, J. (1995). Brazilian congress highlights new directions for epidemiologic methodology. *Epidemiology Monitor, 16,* 6:3, 8.
Longino, C.F., Jr. & Murphy, J.W. (1995). *The old age challenge to the biomedical model: Paradigm strain and health policy.* Amityville, NY: Baywood.
Mann, C.C. (1995). Press coverage: Leaving out the big picture. *Science, 269, July 14:* 166.
Marmot, M., Bobak, M., & Smith, G.D. (1995). Explanations for social inequalities in health. In B.C. Amick III, S. Levine, A.R. Tarlov, & D.C. Walsh (Eds.), *Society and health,* 172-210. New York: Oxford University Press.
Ornish, D. (1992). *Dr. Dean Ornish's program for reversing heart disease.* New York: Ballantine Books.
Overman, S.E. (1989). Continuities in the development of the physical and social sciences: Principles of a new social physics. *Knowledge in Society, 2,* 2:80-93.
Pearce, N. (1996). Traditional epidemiology, modern epidemiology, and public health. *American Journal of Public Health, 86,* 5:678-683.
Rogers, E.M. (1976). Communication and development: The passing of the dominant paradigm. In E.M. Rogers (Ed.), *Communication and development* (pp. 121-148). Beverly Hills, CA: Sage.
Susser, M. & Susser, E. (1996). Choosing a future for epidemiology: I. Eras and paradigms. *American Journal of Public Health, 86,* 5:668-673.
Susser, M. & Susser, E. (1996). Choosing a future for epidemiology: II. From black box to Chinese boxes and eco-epidemiology. *American Journal of Public Health, 86,* 5:674-677.
Taubes, G. (1995). Epidemiology faces its limits. *Science, 269:*164-169.

Vernberg, D. & Murphy, J. (1996). Perceived risk, knowledge, and the lifeworld. In A-T Tymieniecka (Ed.), *Analecta Husserlina*, Vol. 48 (pp. 121-134). Dordrecht: Kluwer Academic Publishers.

Wartenberg, D. & Simon, R. (1995). Integrating epidemiologic data into risk assessment. *American Journal of Public Health, 85,* 4:491-493.

Wilkinson, R. (1992). National mortality rates: The impact of inequality. *American Journal of Public Health, 82*:1082-1084.

A World View Model
of Health Care Utilization:
The Impact of Social and Provider Context
on Health Care Decision-Making

James G. Daley, PhD
Deborah J. Bostock, MD

SUMMARY. This article provides a conceptual model illustrating the filtering effect that social factors have on a health care event. Individual, family and social network filters translate the symptom for the patient before and after s/he enters the health care delivery system. Simultaneously, managed care and provider filters shape what resource is provided by the health care provider to the patient. Basic premises are that decision-making about health care utilization is a complex social interaction and that better attention to the social context will increase the likelihood of effective health care occurring. *[Article copies available for a fee from The Haworth Document Delivery Service: 1-800-342-9678. E-mail address: getinfo@haworth.com]*

James G. Daley is Assistant Professor at the School of Social Work, Southwest Missouri State University, Springfield, MO 65804. Deborah J. Bostock is on the faculty at the Family Practice Residency Program, United States Air Force Medical Center, Travis Air Force Base, CA 94535.

The views expressed in this material are those of the authors, and do not reflect the official policy or position of the U.S. government, the Department of Defense, or the Department of the Air Force.

[Haworth co-indexing entry note]: "A World View Model of Health Care Utilization: The Impact of Social and Provider Context on Health Care Decision-Making." Daley, James G., and Deborah J. Bostock. Co-published simultaneously in *Journal of Health & Social Policy* (The Haworth Press, Inc.) Vol. 9, No. 4, 1998, pp. 67-82; and: *Reason and Rationality in Health and Human Services Delivery* (ed: John T. Pardeck, Charles F. Longino, Jr., and John W. Murphy) The Haworth Press, Inc., 1998, pp. 67-82. Single or multiple copies of this article are available for a fee from The Haworth Document Delivery Service [1-800-342-9678, 9:00 a.m. - 5:00 p.m. (EST). E-mail address: getinfo@haworth.com].

INTRODUCTION

This article provides a conceptual framework for understanding how forces impact the patient and provider and how those forces shape the health care event (the doctor's appointment). Its basic premises are that decision-making about health care utilization is a complex social interaction and that better attention to the social context will increase the likelihood of effective health care occurring.

Scanning the literature, the reader finds many explanatory models which describe an aspect of health care decision-making. Current models include such issues as the importance of the patient's perception of the symptom (Beck, 1963; Ellis, 1969), the patient's readiness for change (Prochaska, 1991), the role of the family in health care decisions (McCubbin & Patterson, 1982; Reiss, 1987), the influence of a patient's social network (Lubben, 1988), the "fit" between health care provider and the patient (Bush, Cherkin, & Barlow, 1993), and the impact of managed care on the health care industry (Schultz, Scheckler, Girard, & Barker, 1990). Each perspective emphasizes an important issue but does seem to illustrate only one aspect of a more holistic issue. Additionally, this article seeks to combine elements from several approaches to encourage the consideration of a larger context when health care decisions are made.

We believe that, to understand the context of health care decisions, one must appreciate the rapidly changing health care industry. Therefore, we begin the article with an overview of today's health care arena. Then, we discuss the different components of the world view model. Finally, we discuss implications of the model and future directions.

TODAY'S CONTEXT FOR HEALTH CARE DELIVERY

The Provider's Perspective

Providers of care are bombarded by social forces seeking to mold their health care decision-making (Brown, 1994; Kongstvedt, 1993; Paulson, 1996; Schulz, Scheckler, Girard, & Barker, 1990). The economics of health care is shifting from fee-for-service to managed care organizations. The art of medicine has become the business of medicine. Even the taxonomy of medical care has changed: Physicians become "primary care managers," patients become "consumers," and "illnesses" become episodes of care. Business case analysis is spoken in the same breath as patient care. Defensive medicine becomes a reality as tort reform is argued and discussed.

Elaborate and increasingly cost-containing mechanisms are being developed which seek to oversee all aspects of health care (Culley, 1994; Hurley, Gage, & Freund, 1991). Differences between for-profit and not-for-profit management strategies are melding into a generic model of cost containment (Herrick, 1993; Hillman, Goldfarb, Eisenberg, & Kelley, 1991; Temple & Kron, 1989-90; Warren, 1995; Zarabozo & LeMasurier, 1993). Private industries are astutely looking to negotiate benefits packages which maximize financial responsibility of physicians while minimizing the cost risk to the company (Alkire & Stolz, 1993; Herrle, 1993). Concurrently, private industries are demanding time-limited and cost-efficient outcomes and looking for undesirable provider attitudes through profiling (Frankel, 1992; Kunnes, 1992; Warden, 1994).

As external customers demand change in health care, providers also seek, or are being forced into, changes in how they provide care. The traditional approach of physician as omnipotent chief of a team of physician extenders has evolved into an increasingly egalitarian team approach. Physicians who became accustomed to paternalistic relationships with their patients now are expected to be "team players" with those patients. Patients who have placed their physicians on pedestals in their communities are now part of the health care team along with nurses, physician assistants, case managers, and other health care providers. Independent status is now possible for nurse practitioners, physician assistants and physical therapists. Psychologists can autonomously prescribe medication in some states. Social workers can obtain insurance reimbursement autonomous of physician co-signature. Physician decisions are being evaluated by long-distance, non-physician case managers before insurance reimbursement is authorized. Efforts are increasing to utilize "decision support" strategies which contrast provider decision-making to computer-based, real-time models of "best" strategies (Gray & Glazer, 1994). In sum, the health care delivery system is evolving and providers are stunned by the change.

As the health care approach transforms, efforts to adapt are rampant. Providers-in-training are being educated about managed care strategies with the hope of shaping the fiscally focused provider of tomorrow (Beigel & Santiago, 1995; Reid, Hosteltler, Webb, & Cimino, 1995; Starfield, 1993; Strom-Gottfried, 1997). Tips abound for current providers on how to survive the managed care tsunami (Appelbaum, 1993; Dorwart, 1990; Feldman, 1992; Hersch, 1995; Kongstvedt, 1993; Mizrahi, 1993) and provide ethical care (Sabin, 1994). Subspecialists are scrambling for security in a rapidly changing world of gatekeeper mentality (Ringel, 1993; Rivo, 1993). And critics challenge that the losses outweigh the gains with this emerging new arena of health care (Bennett, 1993; Giles, 1991; Hunter, 1992; Rodriguez, 1989).

The Patient's Perspective

As health care providers reel with change, the patients and their families struggle with a complex, gap-filled health care delivery system. Empowerment in the selection of a "primary care provider" is balanced with more limited access, case management oversight, and rising deductible cost-sharing. Emphasis on prevention and early intervention is increasing but still primarily at the individual level (Schauffler & Rodriguez, 1993). Shorter hospital stays, contrasts between the actual medical bill and "reasonable charges" coverage, and "pre-existing" condition clauses accelerate patient anxiety about seeking a doctor's appointment. Medicaid coverage is constricting, becoming time-limited and tied to politically motivated employability criteria (Warren, 1995).

Facing a medical concern (e.g., chest pain, suspicion of pregnancy, overweight), the patient must make sense of the concern and decide whether to seek provider assistance. Concurrently, the provider and medical care resources have sought to make sense about which concerns to prioritize (e.g., prenatal care, acute medical emergencies, hypertension) and how to best provide access for services (e.g., nurse call-in service, satellite clinics, tertiary care hospital). Several key influences shape how these two components (patient and provider) connect. The world view model of health care utilization seeks to describe these influences.

THE WORLD VIEW MODEL OF HEALTH CARE UTILIZATION

An Overview

The basic premise of this model is that multiple filters impact both patient and health care provider and shape the type of health care event which occurs. Thus the view of the world is seen through the filters. Figure 1 captures the different social filters which transform the original patient symptom and an "ideal" medical resource into mutually modified forces colliding to create health care utilization.

The patient makes sense of the symptom (ranging from acute chest pain to the value of diet change) through a series of interactions with self, family and social network. Before calling the emergency room or primary care clinic, the patient defines and prioritizes the health care issue into an

FIGURE 1. World View Model of Health Care Utilization

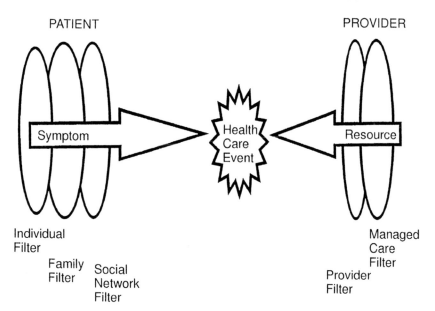

PATIENT   PROVIDER

Symptom

Health Care Event

Resource

Individual Filter

Family Filter   Social Network Filter

Managed Care Filter

Provider Filter

initial context by processing the concern at three levels of feedback (self, family, and network). Let's take an example of a patient with chest pain.

A person wakes up in the middle of the night with a sensation of heaviness on his chest. Does he deny the symptom or grow alarmed? Does he process the symptom with his spouse? Does his spouse minimize or escalate the issue? Does he seek a "second opinion" from his friends or co-workers the next day? Do they minimize or escalate the issue? All these interactions can occur before the first contact with the formal health care system. Symptoms are discussed, worried about, and discarded several times before the patient picks up the phone to set in motion the health care mechanism.

Likewise, the health care resources which the patient seeks have gone through significant fiscal and social processes to produce the service which reacts to his presenting complaint. Before seeing the patient, the health care provider defines and prioritizes the resources available to the patient by responding to the view of managed care and his/her own world view.

For example, a scenario showing the behind-the-scenes evolution of service delivery might be as follows. The family physician's office is converted into a walk-in clinic with a nurse practitioner providing all screening interviews and some of the ongoing care. Hours of operation are cut back. The HMO organization has recently added two more companies with 2,000 covered lives added to the pool of eligible beneficiaries. The emergency resources are cut back with all emergencies being referred to the one remaining community hospital emergency room. EKG equipment is not available at the walk-in clinic; EKGs now routinely take three weeks to schedule. The primary care physician has three examination rooms and has patients scheduled at five-minute intervals. The physician relies heavily on the nursing staff for screening, initial history taking, and following up with the physician's orders. The nurse practitioner summarizes each case in the hall before the physician enters the patient's examination room.

Speed, efficiency, and rapid diagnosis are essential to maintaining the flow of the provider's office. All staff are acutely aware that their decisions are being tracked and profiled against "typical" decisions by similar providers. Volume of patients seen, frequency of diagnostic tests or subspecialty consultations ordered, and costliness of medications (e.g., generic versus name brand) are being tracked with "report cards" reviewed by HMO administration.

Now add the patient to this scenario. The hesitant, fearful patient with unclear symptoms colliding with the speed-obsessed medical staff can lead to escalating frustration in both patient and provider. The provider seeks to give the patient the illusion of a relaxed, casual office visit where the patient's needs are paramount and nothing is rushed. Behind the illusion is a harried provider trying to get to the "bottom line" and leave. The patient seeks to be helpful and concise but carries into the examination room all the internal fears and social misinformation which precedes the office visit.

This interactive process is rarely captured in today's managed care data on access, volume of diagnostic categories seen, or provider profiling. The value of a world view impact model can be to emphasize the interactive context surrounding that managed care data set.

THE PATIENT FILTER

To understand the world view model, we begin with understanding the "filters" which modify the initial symptom of the patient. Before seeking the opinion of others regarding a health care concern, the patient first makes sense of the issue within his own world view. This internal world view is based on four key factors: Perception, Readiness for Change,

Internal Resources, and Illness Experiences (PRII). These factors combine to produce the view of the symptom or concern which is to be shared with significant others.

The Patient's Perception

The fact that a person's perception colors his reaction to an event is not a new concept. Behavioral-cognitive approaches (e.g., Beck, 1963; Ellis, 1969) have long advocated that cognitive perspectives are essential to changing patient behavior. Studies have shown that the way the patient presents the complaint can directly affect the provider's approach to the problem (Birdwell, Herbers, & Kroenke, 1993). Several models have already included patient perception as a key component (McCubbin & Thompson, 1991; Reiss, 1987). The world view model draws heavily from one model in particular, McCubbin's Double ABCX Model. McCubbin, building on Hill's earlier ABCX model (Hill, 1949), describes how a family's perception, resources, and amount of stressors are part of what changes a stressor into a crisis. The model works equally well with individuals as with families.

According to McCubbin's model, a patient's optimistic perception is an essential though not complete factor differentiating between successful or unsuccessful adaptation to a medical stressor. In other words, perception serves as a filter between the stressor (e.g., a child's high fever) and how much the stressor is seen as a medical problem (e.g., rushing the child to the emergency room versus giving the child aspirin and observing). Effective work with changing the perception of the event has often been shown to result in improved treatment cooperation (McCubbin & Patterson, 1982).

Patient's Readiness for Change

Readiness for change is most often shown as a model of progressive willingness to change health damaging behaviors (Prochaska, 1991). Readiness sequences from (a) unwilling to change, (b) slight interest, (c) ambivalent, (d) willing to change, and (e) committed to change. Prochaska's model has included some initial scale development to help with assessing the "stage of readiness" of a patient and tying the readiness stage to the type of intervention attempted (Davidson, 1992; McConnaughy, DiClemente, Prochaska, & Vilicer, 1989; Prochaska & Goldstein, 1991). Thus, a tobacco user with chronic obstructive pulmonary disease in an unwilling stage would get a different approach on smoking cessation than a tobacco user in a committed stage. The importance of this aspect is that understanding how willing a patient is to deal with a symptom can help the provider focus their intervention. There has been no research done looking at the readiness for change of the provider or the cumulative readiness for change of the family unit.

Internal Resources of the Patient

The "internal resources" (a term used in McCubbin's ABCX Model) impact how well a patient reacts to a health concern. Resources can include physical (amount of sleep, exercise frequency, dietary regularity), emotional (affective capability, frequency of sharing concerns with others), and cognitive (dissonance, negative thinking habits). As the internal resources deplete, the resilience of the individual decreases. When facing a significant stressor (e.g., possible diagnosis of cancer), many people will sleep poorly, eat irregularly, decrease exercise, bottle-up affect, and/or think often about the worst possible outcome. McCubbin's point is that these activities reduce the coping capability of the patient and impact on decision-making regarding health care needs. If the internal resources decrease enough, the stressor can become a crisis simply because the patient doesn't feel capable of dealing with the issue any longer. Therefore, the patient phones the on-call physician at 3 a.m. to complain about a headache of five days duration. The physician is puzzled about why the patient went into crisis at 3 a.m. The answer is most likely the internal resources were finally depleted to a low enough level to prompt action.

Patient's Illness Experiences

Past experiences with illness also define the patient's world view. Chest pain is conceptualized differently within a patient whose father died of an acute heart attack than within a patient with no family history of heart disease. A patient who perceived indifferent medical care in the last three clinic visits will react quite differently than a patient satisfied with previous clinic contacts. Past experiences define what the patient will expect if this symptom results in a clinic visit.

THE FAMILY FILTER

As the patient is making sense of the health care concern, the family is often the first and sometimes most potent interpreter of health care need

(House, Landis, & Umberson, 1988). Most simply, significant others are initial sounding boards which can either amplify or defuse the urgency of a symptom. A child with acute abdominal pain can prompt either an emergency room visit or a home remedy depending on the world view of the family.

Importance of Family's Perception

Beyond being a sounding board, the family is the perceptual compass for the patient. Family units "construct reality" and the family's "construction of reality" sets the parameters for family members' behavior (Reiss, 1987). If the health concern is congruent with family beliefs, the patient pursues provider care. If family beliefs forbid provider involvement, the patient will seek solutions only within the family resources. Thus, a kidney dialysis patient is violently ill during weekly dialysis but disregards efforts to change the diet from established family cooking habits. The choice is alliance with family over physical comfort or improved health status.

Family's Interaction Style

In addition to family perceptions, family interaction styles dictate how the initial symptom is filtered through the family unit. Cohesion, flexibility, and communication styles within a family set parameters about how the patient processes his or her concerns (Olson, Sprenkle, & Russell, 1979; Olson, McCubbin, Barnes, Larsen, Muxen, Wilson, 1983). Rigid, distant families dictate minimal openness about family member concerns; flexible, close families encourage open dialogues. The type of family interaction provides either a conduit or barrier to leading the patient to bring the symptom to a health care provider.

Concurrently, family interaction helps shape the symptom into a family-level view of the concern. For example, the chest pain patient discusses the primary symptom; family members suggest that "you just ate too much last night" and the issue is redefined as indigestion. The chest pain patient now seeks help with indigestion.

In sum, the family adds to the patient's own perceptions of the symptom by filtering the issue through their own perspectives. Often, the presenting diagnosis and action plan are agreed upon within the family. After the doctor's visit, the provider's decisions are reprocessed and translated into a family-acceptable paradigm.

THE SOCIAL NETWORK FILTER

Social Network as Interpreter

Frequently the patient also discusses health concerns with friends and trusted colleagues both before and after a health care event. Whether as comparison or confirmation of a personal or family view, the social network of the patient translates the symptom into another layer of interpretation. The patient's view of chest pain versus indigestion adds other views of illness experiences, fears about medical quackery, and suggestions on when and where to seek medical care. Conversely, sometimes the social network can challenge a family assessment of the problem and get the patient to reconsider another explanation.

In a case known to one of these authors, an industrial setting supervisor (with a previous history of two myocardial infarctions [heart attacks]) had three days of chest pain. Despite the discomfort, the supervisor still went to work because the shifts were short-staffed. When he arrived, he mentioned the heaviness sensation to a co-worker who alerted the safety supervisor. The safety supervisor spent more than an hour negotiating with the patient to seek medical attention, including contacting the physician and passing on the doctor's concurrence that immediate medical assessment was essential. When the patient was evaluated, he was immediately placed in an intensive care unit. The social network served effectively as an informal triage unit for the physician.

Linkage of Social Network to Family

Often the degree of importance of the social network is inverse to the importance of the family's input. Enmeshed families produce rigid boundaries and significant limitations to extra-familial sharing; more porous families have stronger external bonds with social networks (Olson et al., 1983; Minuchin, 1974). As the connectedness increases, the influx of social world views increases.

THE HEALTH CARE PROVIDER FILTER

While the patient's interpretation of the symptom is socially congealing, the medical resources available to the patient are modified by both the provider's view and the organizational view. The world view of the provider combines the provider's perspective (created by such factors as perception, interaction style, experiences, and current capability), and the influence of the managed care environment.

The Provider's Perspective

Each provider brings a philosophy to the health care contact. Do people or disease state the focus of the provider? Does a patient's psychosocial concerns prompt curiosity or irritation? Providers decide whether the patient or fiscal coverage dictate the care offered. Providers tend to choose their specialty according to the fit with their personality and view of how they want to fit in the medical arena (Taylor, 1993). Their training reinforces the philosophies inherent in the specialty. Therefore, before they have met the patient, providers have a view of how the patient care should be provided and what is or is not within their area of expertise.

Confidence in one's own abilities to practice a certain aspect of medicine will also impact the view of the provider. Bush, Cherkin, and Barlow showed that "providers who have more confidence in their abilities to effectively manage low back pain may in fact be more effective patient educators" (1993, p. 301). Providers who effectively educate their patients can more effectively impact upon the patient's world view of medicine.

Provider experiences also shape his world view. A difficult residency rotation on cardiology, previous complications with homeless alcoholics, chastisement by senior staff for ordering "too many" tests, and many other events meld the provider's experiences into habits of medical practice. Concurrently, the volume of experience dictates the comfort level and security of the provider.

Finally, the provider brings his current physical and emotional state into the initial contact with the patient. An appointment early in the day can prompt a different reaction than an appointment late in the day when the provider is already 45 minutes behind, tired, and concerned about previous patients seen. Finishing a 26-hour shift, distracted by a beeper going off, and aware that chart dictation is lagging behind, the resident will be struggling to hear clearly the patient describe chronic, vague headaches.

In sum, a combination of several factors culminates in how the provider approaches the health care appointment. However, the managed care philosophy also influences the provider and the setting available to provide health care.

THE MANAGED CARE FILTER

In today's medical arena, there is always an unwelcome voyeur of the medical care episode: the managed care infrastructure. Managed care advocates have potently shaped what resource is available to the patient. Examples include reprioritizing and rationing of health care reimbursement, profiling and impacting provider decision-making, structural limitation on access (e.g., closing of emergency rooms, OB coverage), appointment times (e.g., time slots for appointments and amount of appointments available for provider), screening processes (e.g., beginning of nurse screeners, reimbursement case managers), and staffing levels (e.g., downsizing, changes of training qualifications for support staff).

In the vigorous effort to stabilize rising costs, the world view of the managed care establishment has dramatically reset parameters of available choices before the patient enters the clinic. Patients have to navigate through required primary care managers, pre-approval of outpatient procedures, preferred lists of providers, pharmacies, and other health care resources in a paperwork jungle.

A more extensive discussion of the managed care arena is in the earlier section of this article "Today's Context for Health Care Delivery." The main point is that providers bring into the examination room a myriad of managed care governors which partially dictate the path the health care event will take.

CONCLUSION

Today's managed care agenda dictates better care at the cheapest cost. However, the focus is on tracking the health care utilization without acknowledging the potent impact of multiple social filters regarding how the patient utilizes the health care resources. This article has conceptualized a model which illustrates the contextual factors which drive how the symptom and resources are modified before reaching the health care event.

Health care providers must recognize the filters, and how the different systems translate what the provider intends as medical treatment (including medication usage, diagnostic credibility, and follow-up compliance). In addition, the health care provider should be sensitized to the forces limiting resource choices for the patient. Finally, the health care provider should maintain an awareness of factors impacting his own world view: ideology, experiences, and current conditions.

This model can be invaluable in teaching patients and families about the importance of understanding medical issues. The family is the first social influence on the patient; effective education of the family can impact the likelihood of a patient getting needed care early.

Research is needed to provide empirical evidence of the accuracy and utility of the world view model for health care providers. Research expanding different components of the model (e.g., expanding Prochaska's model to family-level data) would be useful. A path analysis study showing the cumulative effect of each world view on the resulting health care event would be invaluable.

In conclusion, we must look beyond fiscal spreadsheets and high technology assets to truly impact on the health status of patients. The world view model helps remind us that people are the essential links to effective health care.

REFERENCES

Alkire, A.A., & Stolz, S.W. (1993). The employer's view of managed health care: From a passive to an aggressive role. In P.R. Kongstvedt (Ed.), *The managed health care handbook* (2nd ed.) (pp. 255-264). Gaithersburg, MD: Aspen.

Appelbaum, P.S. (1993). Legal liability and managed care. *American Psychologist, 48*(3), 251-257.

Beck, A.T. (1963). Thinking and depression: I. Idiosyncratic content and cognitive distortions. *Archives of General Psychiatry, 9*, 324-333.

Beigel, A., & Santiago, J.M. (1995). Redefining the general psychiatrist: Values, reforms, and issues for psychiatry residency education. *Psychiatric Services, 46*(8): 769-774.

Bennett, M.J. (1993). View from the bridge: Reflections of a recovering staff model HMO psychiatrist. *Psychiatric Quarterly, 64*(1): 45-75.

Birdwell, B.G., Herbers, J.E., & Kroenke, K. (1993). Evaluating chest pain: The patient's presentation style alters the physician's diagnostic approach. *Archives of Internal Medicine, 153*, 1991-1995.

Brown, F. (1994). Resisting the pull of the health insurance tarbaby: An organizational model for surviving managed care. *Clinical Social Work Journal, 22*, 59-71.

Bush, T., Cherkin, D., & Barlow, W. (1993). The impact of physician attitudes on patient satisfaction with care for low back pain. *Archives of Family Medicine, 2*(3), 301-305.

Culley, G.A. (1994). 'Fried chicken' medicine: The business of primary care. *Journal of Family Practice, 38*(1), 68-73.

Davidson, R. (1992). Prochaska and Diclemente's model of change: A case study? *British Journal of Addiction, 87*, 821-822.

Dorwart, R.A. (1990). Managed mental health care: Myths and realities in the 1990s. *Hospital and Community Psychiatry, 41* (10), 1087-1091.

Ellis, A. (1969). A cognitive approach to behavior therapy. *International Journal of Psychotherapy, 8*, 896-900.

Feldman, S. (Ed.). (1992). *Managed mental health services.* Springfield, IL: Charles C Thomas.

Frankel, P.W. (1992). Profiling ambulatory care physicians. *Journal of Health Care Benefits, Nov/Dec*, 21-24.

Giles, T.R. (1991). Managed mental health care and effective psychotherapy: A step in the right direction? *Journal of Behavior Therapy & Experimental Psychiatry, 22* (2), 83-86.

Gray, G.V., & Glazer, W.M. (1994). Psychiatric decision making in the 90's: The coming era of decision support. *Behavioral Healthcare Tomorrow, Jan/Feb,* 47-54.

Herrick, R.R. (1993). Medicaid and managed care. In P.R Kongstvedt (Ed.), *The managed health care handbook* (2nd ed.) (pp. 373-381). Gaithersburg, MD: Aspen.

Herrle, G.N. (1993). Rating and underwriting. In P.R. Kongstvedt (Ed.), *The managed health care handbook* (2nd ed.) (pp. 299-308). Gaithersburg, MD: Aspen.

Hersch, L. (1995). Adapting to health care reform and managed care: Three strategies for survival and growth. *Professional Psychology: Research and Practice, 26,* 16-26.

Hill, R. (1949). *Families under stress: Adjustment to the crises of war separation and reunion.* New York: Harper & Brothers.

Hillman, A.L., Goldfarb, N., Eisenberg, J.M., & Kelley, M.A. (1991). An academic medical center's experience with mandatory managed care for Medicaid recipients. *Academic Medicine, 66*(3), 134-138.

House, J.S., Landis, K.R., & Umberson, D. (1988). Social relationships and health. *Science, 241,* 540-545.

Hunter, D.J. (1992). Doctors as managers: Poachers turned gamekeepers? *Social Science and Medicine, 35*(4), 557-566.

Hurley, R.E., Gage, B.J., & Freund, D.A. (1991). Rollover effects in gatekeeper programs: Cushioning the impact of restricted choice. *Inquiry, 28*(4), 375-384.

Kongstvedt, P.R. (Ed.). (1993). *The managed health care handbook* (2nd ed.). Gaithersburg, MD: Aspen.

Kunnes, R. (1992). Managed mental health: The insurer's perspective. In S. Feldman, (Ed.), *Managed mental health services* (pp. 101-125). Springfield, IL: Charles C Thomas.

Lubben, J. (1988). Assessing social networks among elderly populations. *Family & Community Health, 11*(3), 42-52.

McConnaughy, E.A., DiClemente, C.C., Prochaska, J.O., & Vilicer, W.F. (1989). Stages of change in psychotherapy: A follow-up report. *Psychotherapy, 26*(4), 494-503.

McCubbin, H.I., & Patterson, J.M. (1982). Family adaptation to crises. In H.I. McCubbin, A.E. Cauble, & J.M. Patterson (Eds.), *Family stress, coping, and social support* (pp. 26-47). Springfield, IL: Charles C Thomas.

McCubbin, H., & Thompson, A.L. (Eds.). (1991). *Family assessment inventories for research and practice* (2nd ed.). Madison, WI: University of Wisconsin-Madison.

Minuchin, S. (1974). *Families and family therapy.* Cambridge, MA: Harvard University Press.

Mizrahi, T. (1993). Managed care and managed competition: A primer for social work. *Health & Social Work, 18*(2), 86-91.

Olson, D.H., Sprenkle, D.H., & Russell, C.S. (1979). Circumplex model of marital and family systems I: Cohesion and adaptability dimensions, family types, and clinical applications. *Family Process, 18*, 3-28.

Olson, D.H., McCubbin, H.I., Barnes, H.L., Larsen, A.S., Muxen, M.J., & Wilson, M.A. (1983). *Families: What makes them work.* Beverly Hills, CA: Sage.

Paulson, R.I. (1996). Swimming with the sharks or walking in the garden of Eden? In P.R. Raffoul & C.A. McNeese (Eds.), *Future issues for social work practice* (pp. 85-96). Needham Heights, MA: Allyn & Bacon.

Prochaska, J.O. (1991). Prescribing to the stage and level of phobic patients. *Psychotherapy, 28*(3), 463-468.

Prochaska, J.O., & Goldstein, M.G. (1991). Process of smoking cessation: Implications for clinicians. *Clinics in Chest Medicine, 12*(4), 727-735.

Reid, W.M., Hostetler, R.M., Webb, S.C., & Cimino, P.C. (1995). Time to put managed care into medical and public health education. *Academic Medicine, 70*(8), 662-664.

Reiss, D. (1987). *The family's construction of reality.* Cambridge, MA: Harvard University Press.

Ringel, S.P. (1993). Can neurologists survive or thrive with health care reform? *Annals of Neurology, 33*(5), 441-444.

Rivo, M.L. (1993). Internal medicine and the journey to medical generalism. *Annals of Internal Medicine, 119*(2): 146-152.

Rodriguez, A.R. (1989). Evolutions in utilization and quality management: A crisis for psychiatric services? *General Hospital Psychiatry, 11*(4), 256-263.

Sabin, J.E. (1994). A credo for ethical managed care in mental health practice. *Hospital and Community Psychiatry, 45*(9), 859-861, 869.

Schauffler, H.H., & Rodriguez, T. (1993). Managed care for preventive services: A review of policy options. *Medical Care Review, 50*(2), 153-198.

Schulz, R., Scheckler, W.E., Girard, C., & Barker, K. (1990). Physician adaptation to health maintenance organizations and implications for management. *Health Services Research, 25*(1 pt 1), 43-64.

Starfield, B. (1993). The promise of HMOs: Primary care, prevention, research and education. *HMO Practice, 7*(3), 103-119.

Strom-Gottfried, K. (1997). The implications of managed care for social work education. *Journal of Social Work Education, 33*(1), 7-18.

Taylor, A. (1993). *How to choose a medical specialty* (2nd ed.). Atlanta, GA: Saunders.

Temple, P.C., & Kron, S. (1989-90). The Philadelphia Health Insurance Organization: The results of managed health care for 96,000 medical assistance recipients. *Health Matrix, 7*(4), 12-20.

Warden, G.L. (1994, Sept. 14). Back to the future: Reinventing and integrating behavioral health care. Presented at the National Dialogue Conference on Mental Health Benefits and Practice in the Era of Managed Care. Washington, DC: Behavioral Health Care Tomorrow.

Warren, R.V. (1995). *Merging managed care and medicaid: Private regulation of public health care.* Washington, DC: National Association of Social Workers, Office of Policy and Practice.

Zarabozo, C., & LeMasurier, L. (1993). Medicare and managed care. In P.R. Kongstvedt (Ed.), *The managed health care handbook* (2nd ed.) (pp. 321-344). Gaithersburg, MD: Aspen.

Health Care Policy in Theory and Practice: A Review of the Process as a Product of Rational Decision-Making

Marvin Prosono, PhD

SUMMARY. Decisions are not made in a vacuum. Both theories and practical circumstances influence how reason and decision-making are conceived. In this article, the focus is on organizations and their impact on shaping the decision-making process. Organizational theories, management philosophies, and structural considerations are reviewed, with emphasis placed on how they influence the search for information, the conceptualization of data, the possible uses of knowledge, and the formation of behavioral goals. Accordingly, decision-making is contextualized; organizational assumptions are linked to the reasonableness of a decision. As modern writers say, the "taken-for-grantedness" of an organization is illustrated to be tied inextricably to the nature of reason and assessments of rationality. *[Article copies available for a fee from The Haworth Document Delivery Service: 1-800-342-9678. E-mail address: getinfo@haworth.com]*

INTRODUCTION

As the decade of the 1990s draws to a close, it is a commonplace that American health policy needs serious re-thinking; however, before some-

---

Marvin Prosono is Professor of Sociology at Southwest Missouri State University, Springfield, MO 65804.

[Haworth co-indexing entry note]: "Health Care Policy in Theory and Practice: A Review of the Process as a Product of Rational Decision-Making." Prosono, Marvin. Co-published simultaneously in *Journal of Health & Social Policy* (The Haworth Press, Inc.) Vol. 9, No. 4, 1998, pp. 83-99; and: *Reason and Rationality in Health and Human Services Delivery* (ed: John T. Pardeck, Charles F. Longino, Jr., and John W. Murphy) The Haworth Press, Inc., 1998, pp. 83-99. Single or multiple copies of this article are available for a fee from The Haworth Document Delivery Service [1-800-342-9678, 9:00 a.m. - 5:00 p.m. (EST). E-mail address: getinfo@haworth.com].

thing can be *re*-thought, it has to be the product of thought in the first place. Most analyses of health policy take an unexamined realist position with respect to the generation of policy and the problem(s) with which such policy is meant to contend.

A *realist* position in this context means that those who analyze the generation/implementation/evaluation/culmination of health policy make a number of assumptions, including: (a) social problems are definable; (b) social interests are identifiable; (c) policy makers have adequate information; (d) policy makers have sufficient power; (e) correct policy is attainable; (f) incorrect policy is distinguishable; (g) there is a cause/effect relationship between policies and realities; (h) policy-making is a rational enterprise, among other assumptions.

This paper takes as its purpose a partial review of how health policy is made (or comes into existence) and the implications of that process in a post-modern environment; wherein, it is boldly asserted that social analysis should not be satisfied with relying upon such worn-out academic pieties. Thus, the following is an attempt to de-construct and re-construct the decision-making processes which underlie the production of health policy. First, the very idea of a "health policy" shall be rendered problematic and the organizational and institutional context of its development described; second, four very different historical milestones in the development of health policy shall be briefly considered; and, third, organizational theory is utilized to understand the nature of the American health policy environment, followed by a comment on what may be the limits of the presently constituted system of policy making.

HEALTH POLICY: ENVIRONMENTS AND DECISIONS

The Problem

One of the most perplexing and complex features of life in a democratic society is the construction of policy. How it is made ranks with the two other things deemed best not to know–how laws and sausages are made. It is a messy business and the ingredients are not always so appetizing. The question of health policy has taken on an enormous importance. According to estimates from the Congressional Budget Office, the United States will spend 18.9% of the Gross Domestic Product on health care by the year 2000 (*The President's Health Security Plan*, 1993, p. 284). Although the rate of growth in the health care budget may be leveling off or even decreasing, the U.S. continues to spend far in excess of what any other industrialized nation spends for health care. How is it possible that Japan, which spends approximately 10% of its Gross Domestic Product on health care, is able to provide care for all its citizens? Like so many other nations which spend less than the U.S., Japan has a lower infant mortality rate and a higher life expectancy. These figures, of course, are gross over-simplifications of a very complex health care picture; nonetheless, it is conceded that there is a serious problem which needs to be addressed, questions which need to be answered and decisions which need to be made.[1]

> Sophisticated observers from other nations admire the scientific and technological accomplishments of American medicine but are incredulous that we can expend such vast resources and still have large segments of our population uninsured and underinsured and persistent barriers to offering every person access to basic health care. (Mechanic, 1994, p. 20)

It is not the intention of this paper to grapple with the problem of inequities and irrationalities, but rather to explore the nature and creation of health care policy itself.

An interesting aspect of policy-making is its "taken-for-grantedness," a phenomenon often found when "health policy" becomes the object of study. If health policy is studied as a series of recommendations for optimal decision-making, then such study might be characterized as "normative."[2] Historical studies, international comparative studies, and sociological and economic analyses attempt to place present problems in context so that previous mistakes may be avoided and the problems may be "solved" (Somers & Somers, 1977; Litman & Robins, 1984; Fox, 1986; Shortell & Reinhardt, 1992; Mechanic, 1994; Patel & Rushefsky, 1995).

On the other hand, the study of decision-making can be descriptive (i.e., it may be desirable to explain the behavior of decision-makers rather than enter into the very context of the problem which has been delineated by them). In a sense, this strategy for exploration resembles some of the post-modern and deconstructive work performed by Foucault[3] and others in bringing out the interests and the power which underlie ongoing change in social conditions. Why should we concern ourselves with describing the behavior of the policy/decision-makers rather than assist them with solving their problems? First, by studying the behavior of the policy-makers, it may be possible to avoid becoming suborned by the very definition of the problem (and their place in solving it) advanced by them. Second, it becomes possible to question the nature of policy itself.

The Nature of Policy

The nature of policy is not entirely self-evident. In fact, this concept is so heavily freighted that it is not always certain which one of its many nuances is being employed. In simplest terms, a policy refers to an intended course of action, a planned direction for activity, a line of continuous meaning. As such, it may or may not ever be realized or exercised. For example, during the long years of the Cold War, the United States had a nuclear deterrent policy which seemed to work, but operated as a bluff, prepared for, and supported by, assorted kinds of military and technological hardware. That policy provided a boundary for activity both on the part of our defensive and offensive apparatus and on the part of the apparatus of other nations, friendly and unfriendly.

An entirely different perspective on policy can be discerned by considering health policy and how it is made. To what precisely does health policy refer? It provides both a boundary for activity and a line of action, but it is more than that. Health policy is a signal of intent, a promise to an electorate, a pledge of stability to commercial and professional interests, a predicted outcome as well as the ratification of basic social, political and cultural values. I would argue that the United States has a health policy by default and various observers often read policy back into what was otherwise a less-than-organized period of social action.

An interesting example of attribution of policy by hindsight can be found in Falcone and Hartwig (cited in Litman & Robins, 1984) who discern three periods in American health care history, each focusing on different areas of health policy: 1900-1960, quality of care; 1961-1972, access; 1973-1980, cost-effectiveness. Their analysis makes it appear that there were intentional policy goals which someone was attempting to achieve during those eras; however, this is to find a rational set of policies and goal-oriented behavior during periods when the role of government was not entirely settled, the self-interest of a host of groups was being sorted out, and the institutions necessary to create, implement or enforce policy were either non-existent or in only a nascent stage.

For instance, in discussing the period 1900-1960, Falcone and Hartwig (1984, p. 129) list a number of policy objectives: "upgrade medical education"; "strengthen the scientific basis of medicine"; "upgrade medical practice," etc. This is truly a case of false attribution because the role of government in achieving any of these goals was highly selective or not applicable. It is almost as if to say that whatever line is eventually taken is "policy," that whatever happens is the result of a policy. For any sense at all to be made of the concept of policy, it must be understood as prospective and not as *retrospective*. Policy-makers could never make a false step if whatever happens were to become the, then intended, consequence of the policy read back into a past unable to complain of such self-aggrandizing revisionism.

The development of a rational health care policy has become one of the most difficult challenges with which all levels of government in the United States have had to wrestle at the end of the twentieth century. There have been no end of analyses of, and recommendations for, such policy, especially over the last thirty years. It must be understood at the outset that a short paper cannot possibly review all the myriad attempts to reform or rewrite health care policy made in this country in modern times. What can be done is to establish a framework for understanding the various attempts and why those attempts have either failed or created in their own way further difficulties which then need to be taken into account when (re)formulating health care policy. For that seems to be more the rule than the exception. As each new attempt either succeeds or fails, the "system" becomes more unwieldy and less responsive to any further attempt to get under control what is universally acknowledged to be an unacceptable spiraling of costs accompanied by lower levels of coverage, eroding access and millions left out of the health care loop altogether. How can such a complex and basically rational system of health care lead to such irrational results? Could part of the answer reside in the contradictory and unrealistic demands that are made on the powers of history, government and organization?

American Health Policy Environment

It is here, in discussion of the health policy environment, that the complexities of dealing with any changes in health care become apparent. Again, there are many analyses of the policy environment which round up the usual suspects such as various interest groups or "policy entrepreneurs" (Mueller, 1993). One of the most thorough analyses of health policy environments can be found in Patel and Rushefsky (1995) who detail the political and legal context in which American policy is made. Questions of politics and law are probably most essential.

Because of the peculiar history of American democracy, "health" or "health care" was never mentioned directly in the United States Constitution. The desire of the framers was to reserve all possible powers to the states and the people so that only the nebulous phrase "general welfare" finds a place in that document (Jacobs, 1993). As a result, the history of medical practice and public health in the United States provides an erratic narrative of attempts to organize the provision of health care. What this means for policy-makers on the national level is the lack of a firm basis for taking charge of health care institutions. In a sense, practically all federal involvement in health care is hostage to a patchwork of legislation that can be amended or withdrawn. Often such legislation usually passes with some kind of built-in expiration, resulting, then, in the need for Congressional reapproval of possibly an originally highly contended piece of legislation. All three branches of the federal government may become involved in this health policy tug-of-war.

In addition, the fifty states and many municipalities are also in the health policy business. They provide general hospitals, mental hospitals, and clinics and attempt to coordinate efforts with the federal government which is responsible for financing 42% of all health expenditures. Through its financing, the federal government imposes regulations on the way in which states provide health care to its citizens, especially those citizens who rely on public assistance when seeking access to health care.

After becoming exhausted by attempts to get health care spending under control, as well as provide universal access to health care, states have sought waivers from the Department of Health and Human Services (DHHS) in order to depart from certain regulations and requirements hitherto imposed on them. Such waivers are being granted, permitting health care reform at least to occur on some minimal basis. Oregon was one of the first states to get such a waiver in 1993. In a letter to the then Governor of Oregon, Barbara Roberts, the Secretary of DHHS, Donna Shalala, after congratulating the Governor for initiative and commitment, restated the terms and conditions under which the waiver was being approved:

> These terms are designed to ensure that the plan provides an adequate level of health care services to eligible Medicaid recipients, contains Federal costs, and meets the requirements of the Americans with Disabilities Act. They also guarantee that there will be no change in covered services without prior approval of the Department of Health and Human Services. (Letter of Secretary Shalala, 1993)

This letter exemplifies the control maintained by the federal authorities of state attempts to plot their own health policy course. In this case, the Oregon Plan had to overcome severe criticism for developing a two-tier system of medicine and for rationing health care.

This one contact between the two levels of government emphasizes the enormous complexity involved in coordinating the efforts of the various branches of government, especially when their relations are not constitutionally established in the matter at issue. There is an *ad hoc* quality to the development and management of health care institutions and programs. In addition, interest groups, including, but not limited to, the American Hospital Association, the American Medical Association, the American Association of Retired Persons, American Red Cross, labor unions, and religious denominations create a cacophony of competing voices which renders the formulation of any major overhaul in health care policy problematic. The smaller the attempted modification, or the simpler the adjustment, the more likely a chance it has of succeeding. Any macro-level change, such as that attempted by the Clintons in 1993 (discussed herein) appears doomed to fail.

Finally, the policy environment is also partly a junkyard. It contains the rusting hulks of old, worn-out policies, the discarded ideas, used and unused, of many a think-tank, and the shed skins of government programs outgrown and no longer serviceable. Bureaucracy, operating as the junkyard dog, resists any real change as history, ideology, politics, technology, and market economics taunt it from the other side of the fence. The following historical episodes attempt to demonstrate how health care policy has evolved through time, often escaping the best intentions of policy-makers.

HISTORICAL EPISODES IN THE DEVELOPMENT OF HEALTH POLICY

In order to conduct this survey through time, four episodes have been chosen from the history of health care: (a) Johann Peter Frank and the idea of the medical police in eighteenth-century Germany; (b) Abraham Flexner and the revolution in medical education and practice in early twentieth-century United States; (c) the Hill-Burton Legislation which provided for hospital construction in the late 1940s; and (d) the attempt of the Clinton administration to reform health care in 1993. By briefly considering each of these episodes, the policy environments and contingencies should become apparent.

Johann Peter Frank and the Medical Police

It is interesting to compare the form of health policy in our age with the nascent form it took in Germany before it was unified (pre-1870). It must be remembered that Germany was divided into a number of individual states, many of which were ruled autocratically and whose people were fairly homogeneous with respect to ethnicity, religion and other factors. At the end of the eighteenth century, Johann Peter Frank further developed the idea of the "medical police" which meant that the police power of the state could be mobilized to insure that healthy conditions would prevail with or without the consent of the individual. His six-volume work (the first of which appeared in 1779), describing an entire system of medical police, is a "landmark in the history of thought on the social relations of health and disease" (Rosen, 1974, p. 120). This consisted of attention to living conditions, birth and death rates, the forcible removal of contagions, and, especially, increase in the population. Population increase and the health of workers and soldiers were concerns of particular interest to the various German states.

Another aspect of the policy environment was what came to be called "cameralism," the general perspective which existed within German society on the relations of the people and the state. ". . . [I]t comprised certain ideas of the social relations of individuals and groups, and of the way in which they should be treated in matters of social policy" (Rosen, 1974, p. 122). The health of the population contributed to the ability of the state to play power politics; thus, concern with health became a state matter. An autocratic state, concentrating power in the hands of a few individuals, could achieve certain results in the organization and delivery of health care that could not be achieved in a society in which the health of the population was not defined as so inextricably bound with the fortunes of the state.

Frank had not been the first to recognize the principles necessary to maintain the health of populations, nor was he the last. A number of observers in prior centuries had provided the grounding for state involvement on fundamental Christian values of regard for persons, and the desire to ensure a tranquil and healthy social environment. The Prussian government continued this line well into the nineteenth century and when the germ theory of disease had finally been irrevocably established, the physician Rudolf Virchow[4] played a major part not only in the establishment of public health in his native kingdom, but also in the health of those residents in the whole of Germany. Virchow stated in 1848:

> The democratic state . . . desires that all its citizens enjoy a state of well-being, for it recognizes that they all have equal rights. Since general equality of rights leads to self-government, the state also has the right to hope that everyone will know how through his own labor to achieve and maintain a state of well-being within the limits of the laws set up by the people themselves. However, the conditions of well-being are health and education, so that it is the task of the state to provide on the broadest possible basis the means for maintaining and promoting health and education through public action . . . (Virchow quoted in Rosen, 1974, p. 64)

This statement of health policy is clear and unequivocal. It represents, to a great extent, the attitude toward the provision of health care taken not only by Germany then and today, but also by most of the nations of Europe. What ironically began as a statist view of the importance of health care became the cornerstone of democratic values in a post-autocratic Europe. Thus, such societies do not find it at all problematic to establish health ministries with overarching authority to create and conduct health policy, and they provide interesting comparisons with American market-driven, government-at-arms'-length health care policy.

Abraham Flexner and Reform of Medical Education and Practice

One of the most interesting examples of policy creation can be seen before, during, and after the publication of the Flexner Report. The mature American federal bureaucracy had not yet come into existence, when, in 1910, Abraham Flexner published his survey of all medical schools in the United States and Canada. This report had been prepared at the behest of the Carnegie Foundation for the Advancement of Teaching which had been asked to replicate an earlier study made by the Council on Medical Education of the American Medical Association. Abraham Flexner, a professional educator, personally visited the 155 existing medical schools and described the conditions that he found (Brown, 1979; Ginzburg, 1990).

At the turn of the century, medicine was fast becoming a scientific enterprise and the many medical schools, which had been established on a proprietary basis,[5] requiring little or no prior education from students–nor much in the way of academic mastery in their courses–found themselves unable to compete with the more rigorous and scientifically-oriented institutions. Most of the homeopathic medical schools closed their doors as well as did all but two of the Black medical schools. Flexner had assisted a process already begun and by 1915, ninety-two medical schools had closed their doors or merged. (Brown, 1979, p. 154)

Who had initiated this rather momentous shift in medical education? It had been the General Education Board (the nascent Rockefeller Foundation), the Carnegie Foundation for the Advancement of Teaching and the Council on Medical Education of the American Medical Association. The results of this change in medical education were manifold. Johns Hopkins University Medical School, the first in the United States to require a four-year undergraduate degree for admission, was used as a model. First, the number of physicians was severely reduced because the number of medical schools was reduced; second, the scientific basis of medicine and the research posture of medical education were secured; third, medicine was slowly shifted to hospital-based practice; fourth, specialization was given impetus; fifth, the status of physicians was heightened; sixth, alternative medicine and holistic medicine were placed under severe disabilities, to name but a few of the consequences of the Flexner Report and its associated developments.

How can we explain such momentous change? Where was the locus of decision-making? It certainly was not the government.[6] There was no real government involvement in these changes. Were they rational changes? Inevitable changes? Should the work of Flexner and the various philanthropic and professional organizations on whose behalf he acted be counted as policy-makers? It is ironic that over the past thirty years an expansion in the number of medical schools has again created a "surplus" of physicians, but in the contemporary case, the surplus is in the number of specialists, an attenuated legacy of the Flexner reforms. Efforts are now underway to educate primary care physicians to meet the ever-growing need of a population which is being prepared for a shift into managed care and preventative medicine, a policy choice not necessarily driven by a desire to enhance the health of the populace but to undo the pernicious effects of a health care system which has grown too large, unwieldy and expensive.

The Hill-Burton Act and Hospital Construction

An interesting moment in the development of health policy came shortly after World War II when the Congress passed and President Truman signed the Hill-Burton or Hospital Survey and Construction Act in August 1946. This Act provided grants-in-aid to states so that hospitals could be built in areas that were too poor to afford establishing them, and to increase the number of hospital beds by financing the expansion of existing hospitals.

> The act was designed to be a federal-state partnership, with the federal government providing grants to assist states in inventorying their existing hospitals; surveying the need for the construction of public and nonprofit hospitals; and constructing public and nonprofit hospitals in accordance with the programs developed by the states . . . By the time the program expired in the late 1970s, it had provided $4 billion in grants to nearly 4,000 hospitals and $1.9 billion in loans and loan guarantees to almost 300 hospitals. (Quoting Kenneth Williamson, American Hospital Association representative in Weeks and Berman, 1985, p. 45)

The Act was the result of intense lobbying and consensus building by a coalition of rather diverse interests. At the end of World War II, the federal government had become responsible for the health care of a large number of people including war veterans and their dependents. At the same time, the Flexner reforms had had another generation to deepen their impact. The physicians who had gone to war were a generation with a great deal of scientific expertise. They expected that they would go into group practice after the war and would specialize. The war also spurred federal subsidization of medical education to produce the necessary physicians for the war effort. In addition, the Depression of the 1930s caused major difficulties for the proper funding of existing hospitals or the building of needed facilities.

Nonetheless, there were many groups that had to be convinced that federal financing of hospital construction was not going to undermine physician autonomy, lead to the reorganization of medical practice, or interfere with the traditional role that the states were given by the Constitution. Conservative senators, such as Robert Taft of Ohio, made sure that the bill contained provision for the enshrinement of "local responsibility."[7] In fact, there had been a movement afoot by the Public Health Service and certain foundations to use the occasion of this hospital finance legislation to interpose a new perspective on American health care.

"During the war, philanthropic foundations and the United States Public Health Service helped to establish local coalitions of individuals committed to organizing medical care in regional hierarchies based on hospitals" (Fox, 1986, p. 119). Many groups in the nation including labor unions, liberals and bureaucrats wanted to see a national system of health insurance enacted. Other interest groups such as the Public Health Service and the American Hospital Association believed that regionalization, linking district hospitals with larger university teaching hospitals, was the most effective way of organizing services (Fox, 1986, p. 124). The bill that finally passed contained the provisions which answered conservative concerns, making no attempt to threaten the system of health care delivery then in place. There is an irony when considering that almost fifty years later the administration of President Clinton would propose a health care plan which contained provisions similar to those broached during the debate over Hill-Burton.

President Clinton's Health Reform

One of the major priorities set by the first Clinton administration was a major reform of health care delivery and financing. To this end, President Clinton empowered his wife, Hillary, to establish a panel of experts so as to create the basis for serious health care reform. Before, during, and after the fact, Mrs. Clinton and Ira Magaziner came under serious attack not only for the final details of the health care plan but also for the manner in which it was generated.

> A brain trust presided over by Ira C. Magaziner, the first couple's longtime friend and management whiz, worked in secret on the nitty-gritty, for a time assembling some 500 experts who labored night and day to clarify alternatives and spell out details. (*The President's Health Security Plan*, 1993, p. ix)

The plan began by setting out the problem in a way with which few, if any, could take exception: Americans lack health care security; costs are rising faster than the economy grows; bureaucracy confounds consumers; quality is uncertain; long-term care coverage is inadequate; quality care is out of reach for many; fraud and abuse undermine care (*President's Health Security Plan*, 1993, pp. 3-4). The "Plan," not easily summarized, then went into enormous detail, attempting to solve all the perceived problems in one mighty exertion. Unfortunately, the rest of the country was not up to the effort and the Plan failed to pass Congress; it may have been responsible in part for the enormous electoral losses suffered by the Democratic Party in the 1994 elections.

What did this Plan contain that pushed so many hot-buttons? First, criticism arose over the manner in which the Plan was generated. The secretiveness of meetings and the choice of participants got the process off on the wrong foot. A federal judge eventually ruled that Mrs. Clinton violated federal law by withholding the records of the meetings. Second, the Plan attempted to rework almost the entire health care apparatus. It meant to solve the problems of universal access and runaway costs at the same time, while providing what it called a "Guaranteed National Benefit Package." Third, it involved what appeared to be the rationing of medical care. This seemed inevitable considering that the plan contained a new system of price controls. These controls represented some of the most threatening provisions, which criminalized any physician who attempted to collect fees outside those set by the newly contemplated health alliances. Fourth, entirely new layers of bureaucracy were being proposed— health alliances and regional boards, all controlled by a federal Health Care Board. There were to be a series of other boards created under this central board such as the National Quality Management Program which were to "develop a core set of measures of performance that apply to all health plans, institutions and practitioners" (*President's Health Security Plan*, 1993, p. 113).

This severe federalization of one-seventh of the American economy ignored the basic structures which had grown into place over decades and centuries. It was as if the entire health care apparatus were being designed from the ground up with little or no consideration for, among other things, market forces, insurance and pharmaceutical interests, physician uneasiness with loss of professional autonomy, consumer fear of loss of physician choice and sufficient coverage, and the concern of the elderly with continuity and choice of care. The plan was defeated in Congress and very little, if any, progress has been made by either the executive or legislative branches of government since then in grappling with the problems of health care in general or the Medicare program in particular.

The defeat of the Clinton health reform plan might be attributed to the fact that it was overly ambitious or that it fell victim to the party politics of the moment, or the institutions were resistant to such change (Steinmo & Watts, 1995), or that the class structure mitigated against it (Navarro, 1995). Such explanations do not provide a sufficient explanation of its defeat. The Flexner reforms were certainly as momentous, but they were not governmental reforms. Emanating from professional and commercial interests, these reforms were undertaken in an age when the idea of science swept all before it. There was no way to prevent the medical schools of that age from having to accommodate that scientific ethos. No such dynamic provided the Clinton health reform with the power to succeed. What may further explain this defeat is the organizational and systemic realities of the policy environment.

ORGANIZATIONAL THEORY
AND THE POLICY ENVIRONMENT

Scott (1992) describes three types of organizations. *Rational* organizations " . . . are instruments designed to attain specific goals" (Scott, 1992, p. 29). *Open* organizations are cybernetic in their functioning and respond to the inputs of information which then condition the further operation of the organization. *Natural* organizations are interpreted as, first and foremost, collectivities of human beings, but collectivities which involve informal structure and goal complexity. When considering the emergence of health policy, these forms of organization provide useful models for understanding the role of policy and policy-maker in the larger social setting. Such a use of these organizational models may be stretching their original purpose. They are meant to describe and explain the operation of organizations, but they may also work when considering policy environments. What can they tell us about the way that policy comes into existence?

In the rational model, goals are formalized and the means/ends problem is elaborately worked out. It is expected that roles and functions exist in order to accomplish the goals and if they do not, then they must be created. Bureaucracy most closely fits this model with its hierarchy of offices, division of labor, rules, technical qualification of personnel, etc. Early health policy reflects this bias. Both the example of Johann Peter Frank and Abraham Flexner demonstrate this quality of rationalization as applied to the health scene. There is little attention paid to obtaining consensus since the rational environment itself accepts the policy as formed without necessity to inform or persuade constituencies.

Alternatively, the open policy environment accepts the necessity of both providing and obtaining as much information as possible so that policy will be carefully grounded in the mechanism for which it was designed. The provision of information, the cybernetic effect of feedback, can be complicated by the existence of uncertainty. In a paper which focused upon the organization of medical education, Fox (1957) described three types of uncertainty with which physicians must contend as they make their way through medical school and into medical practice. The first type represents the uncertainty which results from incomplete assimilation of the knowledge available. The second type of uncertainty stems from the incompleteness of medical knowledge at any particular time. Finally, the third type results from the difficulty of distinguishing between the other two types. Does the physician have sufficient knowledge or is there knowledge to be had at all?

In a very real sense, those responsible for the development of policy must contend with these three types of uncertainty. As physicians must understand the etiology of disease, perform correct diagnosis and then provide a prognosis, the policymaker must also understand the background of a problem, be able to identify the nature of the problem and assign some outcome both for the consequences of doing nothing and for intervening. (In the modern, bureaucratic state, there is little likelihood that doing nothing represents a situationally viable option. The "Do No Harm" of medicine finds little parallel in policy making.) Uncertainty dogs the steps of problem-solvers in both cases every step of the way.

Open systems can be further understood using contingency theory whose ". . . general orienting hypothesis [is] that organizations whose internal features best match the demands of their environments will achieve the best adaptation" (Scott, 1992, p. 89). The Hill-Burton Act exemplifies this idea of a policy which is instituted in order to provide feedback so that action might be taken to remedy a possible social problem. States were to survey their stock of hospitals and hospital beds to determine what was needed. Theoretically, once the need was met, the system would react and cease to build hospitals or to increase the number of beds. The Act took into account concerns of various interest groups and won the consent of a diverse group of political and technical figures. It met the demand of the environment. Contrast the Hill-Burton Act with the Clinton health care reform plan and immediately it is apparent that the Clinton plan itself was drafted without an "open" flow of information. The panel charged with its creation did not allow the many constituencies which would be necessary for its passage to have input in its design, compromising its chances from the start.

Finally, the natural systems model appears to represent many of the aspects of the American policy environment. There is a great deal of goal complexity when one considers the enormous economic, political, social and cultural elements involved in the provision of health care. In as open and free a democratic society as exists in the United States, predicated on a legal rather than a traditional basis, it becomes a serious challenge to reform anything, let alone the gargantua which is health care. There are formal and informal structures which preserve and extend the meaning that individuals take from participating in the system. When the Clintons proposed their health care plan, they were apparently in earnest when they attempted to bring almost every aspect of the health care picture into the orbit of a newly minted policy. "To administer a social organization according to purely technical criteria of rationality is irrational, because it ignores the nonrational aspects of social conduct" (Peter M. Blau quoted in Scott, 1992, p. 51).

It may very well be that reform of the *health care system* has such a difficult time in the United States because it is seen as reform of "the system" and not necessarily of health care. *Health care* is often interpreted as an opening wild-eyed reformers are utilizing in order to make more fundamental changes in the economic and social fabric of the nation, rather than limiting their reforms simply to health care issues. This suspicion only masks what may be at the bottom of the health care dilemma. Individual decisions, decisions taken in micro- or meso-level contexts may be entirely rational. As conditions change, as medical technology improves and complexities are added, as social epidemiology adds new knowledge to the causes and vectors of disease, as political attitudes shift, each of the decisions made in answer to the new problems may be rational. Decision-makers are not asked to solve the most basic policy questions. What right do Americans have to health care? How should health care be financed? What level of health care should be guaranteed to citizens if health care is a right? Without a proper resolution to these and other questions, whatever decisions are taken, however rational, will be provisional and, if the past is any lesson, may only exacerbate the problems of an already overly complex and mismanaged non-system. What is needed is a rational, workable health care policy, crafted to fit within American institutional realities, and one which is able to operate without endless tinkering and legislative meddling. Instead, most "health care policy talk" is health care *reform* policy talk. By reflecting upon the history and development of health care, it may be possible to achieve a new perspective, a perspective which understands that it is not *reform* which is needed but *policy* which is needed. This can only be accomplished if there are people who have sufficient will and understanding. The alternative is to continue in this stalemate wherein the provision of health care is torn between half-hearted government involvement and blind market forces while attempted solutions are mired in an endless cycle of ineffective reform.

NOTES

1. Not everyone believes that health care in the United States is in need of any kind of reform. Fred Barnes, a noted political and cultural commentator, does not believe there is a crisis in health care (1993).

2. Distinction between "normative" and "descriptive" studies of decision-making taken from Taylor, 1965.

3. "The research that I am undertaking here therefore involves a project that is deliberately both historical and critical, in that it is concerned–outside all prescriptive intent–with determining the conditions of possibility of medical experience in modern times" (Foucault, 1973, p. xix).

4. "This awareness of the relations of medicine to social problems, Virchow formulated in the somewhat rhetorical but striking slogan: 'Medicine is a social science, and politics nothing but medicine on a grand scale' " (Rosen, 1974, p. 62).

5. Proprietary medical schools were established as profit-making institutions. They had little, if any, entrance requirements, poor equipment, uninterested lecturers, short courses of study and superficial control of students.

6. Government involvement in the regulation of medical practice was uneven during the nineteenth century. The American Medical Association was founded in 1847 specifically to encourage the states to enact mandatory licensing laws in order to drive the medical "irregulars" out of practice. This was not finally achieved until the end of the century.

7. "Taft reminded his colleagues that the bill forced the states to take responsibility for the rights they cherished by requiring them to license and regulate hospitals in exchange for federal grants" (Fox, 1986, p. 129).

REFERENCES

Barnes, F. (1993). What health care crisis? *The American Spectator,* May.

Bishop, C.E. & Wallack, S.S. (1996). "National health expenditure limits: The case for a global budget process." *The Milbank Quarterly, 74*(3), 361-376.

Brown, E.R. (1979). *Rockefeller medicine men. Medicine and capitalism in America.* Berkeley: University of California Press.

Dougherty, C.J. (1988). *American health care. Realities, rights, and reforms.* New York: Oxford University Press.

Foucault, M. (1973). *The birth of the clinic. An archaeology of medical perception.* New York: Vintage Books.

Fox, D.M. (1986). *Health policies, health politics. The British and American experience 1911-1965.* Princeton, NJ: Princeton University Press.

Ginzburg, E. (1990). *The medical triangle. Physicians, politicians, and the public.* Cambridge, MA: Harvard University Press.

Jacobs, L.R. (1993). Health reform impasse: The politics of American ambivalence toward government. *Journal of Health Politics, Policy and Law, 18*(3), 629-655.

Litman, T.J. & Robins, L.S. (Eds.). (1984). *Health politics and policy.* New York: John Wiley & Sons.

March, J.G. (Ed.). (1965). *Handbook of organizations.* Chicago: Rand McNally & Company.

Mechanic, D. (1994). *Inescapable decisions. The imperatives of health reform.* New Brunswick, NJ: Transaction Pubs.

Mueller, K.J. (1993). *Health care policy in the United States.* Lincoln, NE: University of Nebraska Press.

Navarro, V. (1995). Why Congress did not enact health care reform. *Journal of Health Politics, Policy and Law, 20*(2), 454-462.

Patel, K. & Rushefsky, M.E. (1995). *Health care politics and policy in America.* Armonk, NY: M.E. Sharpe.

Rosen, G. (1974). *From medical police to social medicine: Essays on the history of health care.* New York: Science History.

Scott, W.R. (1992). *Organizations: Rational, natural, and open systems.* Englewood Cliffs, NJ: Prentice Hall.

Shortell, S.M. & Reinhardt, U.E. (Eds.). (1992). *Improving health policy and management. Nine critical research issues for the 1990s.* Ann Arbor, MI: Health Administration Press.

Steinmo, S. & Watts, J. (1995). Why comprehensive national health insurance always fails in America. *Journal of Health Politics, Policy and Law, 20*(2), 329-372.

United States Department of Health and Human Services. (1993, May). Letter of the Secretary to Oregon Governor Barbara Roberts.

Weeks, L.E. & Berman, H.J. *Shapers of American health care policy.* Ann Arbor, MI: Health Administration Press.

White, J. (1995). The horses and the jumps: Comments on the health care reform steeplechase. *Journal of Health Politics, Policy and Law, 20*(2), 373-389.

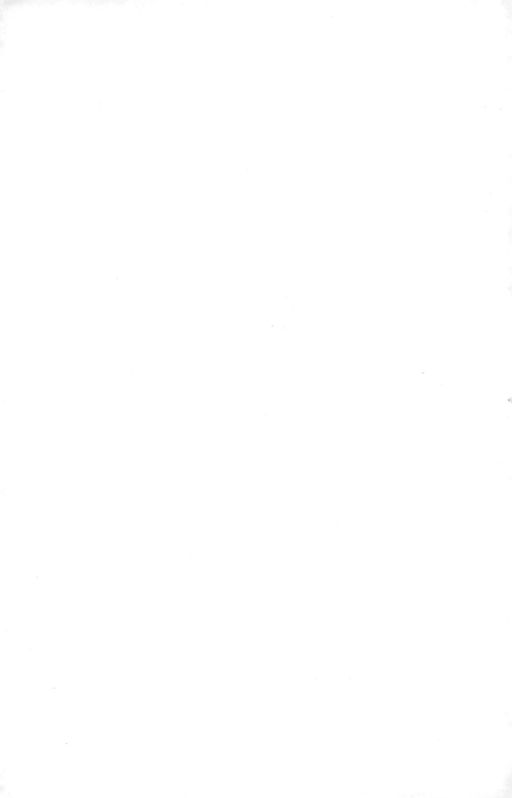

The Limits of Scientific Medicine: Paradigm Strain and Social Policy

Charles F. Longino, Jr., PhD

SUMMARY. In this essay, the historical roots of the dominant medical worldview will be drawn and its tenets will be outlined. The existing paradigm may be called the Western Biomedical Model, whose doctrines include body-mind dualism, physical reductionism, the mechanical analogy, specific etiology and the body as the appropriate focus of regimen and control. Some of the pressures straining the paradigm will be discussed, especially the force of human and population aging and the accompanying dominance of chronic illness as a focus of health care. The tentative outlines of an emergent model will be described in the context of the current health policy debate. The mind, biography, surrounding environment, and culture are a few considerations that become very significant in a non-Cartesian world. *[Article copies available for a fee from The Haworth Document Delivery Service: 1-800-342-9678. E-mail address: getinfo@haworth.com]*

INTRODUCTION

This paper argues that there is a connection between what we think and what we do. What we think begins in a cultural context of ideas and

Charles F. Longino, Jr., is Professor of Sociology and Director of the Reynolda Gerontology Program, Wake Forest University and Associate Director of the Sticht Center, Bowman Gray School of Medicine, Wake Forest University, Winston-Salem, NC 27109.

[Haworth co-indexing entry note]: "The Limits of Scientific Medicine: Paradigm Strain and Social Policy." Longino, Charles F., Jr. Co-published simultaneously in *Journal of Health & Social Policy* (The Haworth Press, Inc.) Vol. 9, No. 4, 1998, pp. 101-116; and: *Reason and Rationality in Health and Human Services Delivery* (ed: John T. Pardeck, Charles F. Longino, Jr., and John W. Murphy) The Haworth Press, Inc., 1998, pp. 101-116. Single or multiple copies of this article are available for a fee from The Haworth Document Delivery Service [1-800-342-9678, 9:00 a.m. - 5:00 p.m. (EST). E-mail address: getinfo@haworth.com].

values that have evolved, often for centuries, and forms the parameters within which policy innovations are made. When cultural paradigms provide the rationale and justification for action, new ways of work become difficult to introduce and to maintain. On the other hand, pressures for policy change tend to strain the existing paradigms. In this essay, the historical roots of the prevailing medical paradigm will be drawn and its tenets will be outlined. Some of the pressures straining the paradigm will be discussed, and the tentative outlines of an emerging paradigm will be described in the context of the current health policy debate.

The existing paradigm may be called the Western biomedical model. This model relies on an understanding of causation, derived from science, that is essentially mechanical. Repairing a body, in this view, is analogous to fixing a machine. Furthermore, this rendition of causation leads to a remarkably optimistic expectation that each disease has a specific cause that is awaiting discovery by medical research. Finally, because the body is the appropriate subject of medical science and practice, this object is also the appropriate subject of regimen and control. These are the doctrines of the biomedical model.

The challenge to this model comes from several sources, including the process of growing older. The aging of the population, including a potential extension of life expectancy, has brought about an increased prevalence of chronic conditions and the deterioration of physiological functioning. But these problems do not have a precise moment of onset, do not have a single and unambiguous cause, do not have an end that can be easily modified, and are implicated in a mélange of factors indirectly related to physiology. Accordingly, the incompatibility between the orthodox medical worldview and the chronic illnesses of members of an aging population is undermining the efficacy of the biomedical model. Yet a paradigm shift–a change in the practical and philosophical worldview–is occurring that will resolve the strain.

In order to comprehend biomedicine properly, the philosophy that sustains the biomedical model must be outlined. Insight is provided in the following section into the key elements of this model. Most important to remember is that dualism is central to the success of orthodox biomedicine.

ROOTS OF THE BIOMEDICAL MODEL

Medicine does not consist simply of the application of sophisticated procedures and techniques. Presupposed by the biomedical model is an image of the individual, valid knowledge, the focus of intervention, causality, and so forth, which are preconditions for the prevailing practice of medicine. A causal historical link cannot be said to exist between these assumptions and the onset of biomedicine (Weber, 1958). Nonetheless, these and other themes support modern medicine.

Certain key philosophical considerations are essential for making sense of how medicine operates as a science. This constellation of ideas might be referred to as the silent side of biomedicine. Foucault, for example, uses the term "episteme" to describe this essential background. An episteme, as he writes, "make[s] possible the appearance of objects during a given period of time" (1989, 33).

Viewed from the cultural position of twentieth century medicine, during early medical history—from the early Greeks to the end of the Medieval Period—any complaint could be the result of a combination of factors, both natural and spiritual. Wholeness included the whole person: the body, mind and spirit. Gradually, the move was away from religion and toward science.

This change did not occur all at once. The admixture of spirit and nature continued until the arrival of Descartes, who wrote in the early 1600s. He made a theoretical maneuver that allowed nature to be "rationalized" (Weber, 1978). Nature, in other words, could be materialized and transformed into an inert object. In this way, facts combined with judicious reasoning could thus be the cornerstone of medicine.

The thrust of Descartes' position is the fact that mind (*res cogito*) could be severed from the body (*res extensa*) (Carlson, 1975). Matter is thus freed from subjectivity; pristine matter is available for inspection. Like nature, the body becomes an object that is encountered. Factors such as mind, soul, consciousness, and spirit, are unimportant and dismissed because of their intangible character. The locus of disease is the body, which is envisioned to be nothing more than a physiological organism.

Following this tactic by Descartes, other changes began to take place that are vital to modern medicine. The belief that facts could be separated categorically from values was spawned. What this meant was that facts were externalized, or thought to be associated with empirical indicators. Physicians could, thus, safely become empiricists and attend solely to physiological markers. How interpretive factors, related to culture or biography, might affect an illness became irrelevant. The experience of persons was denigrated and treated as illusory (Schwartz & Wiggins, 1988). Only "so-called" objective factors were considered real.

Consistent with this transformation of nature, the impetus for action was reformulated as causal. Discussions revolved around "causal chains" and "webs of causation" (Norell, 1984). Adopting this imagery enabled physicians to view events as structurally linked. Accordingly, a sound rationale could be understood to underpin the advent of illness. In this way, the most propitious strategy for intervention could be formulated because causes are predictable and manipulable. Through rigorous research the source of a problem can be pinpointed. Hence, diagnostic activity became a scientific investigative process.

What should be accomplished by a medical intervention was also influenced by the acceptance of either-or, or dualistic, thinking. Sickness or pathology was understood to be a condition of disequilibrium, or of nature out of balance. Restoring the body to "normal" equilibrium became the goal of most interventions. Understanding norms with respect to equilibrium was thought to represent a significant improvement. Abstractions such as the Mean, Middle Way, or Justice (*Dike*) had existed before, but they were abandoned in favor of a more concrete explanation of normativeness. Instead of searching for some primordial guidepost for eternal justice, or Rightness, norms were thought to be inherent in the physiological system and not outside of it. Normativeness and stability were thus not a mythical problem, but a matter of bringing various structures into harmony (Strasser & Randall, 1981). The etiology of imbalance, accordingly, was relatively easy to identify.

A final element of the rational worldview pertains to how knowledge should be acquired. As should be noted, subjectivity or interpretation is a liability in the pursuit of valid data. In order to curtail the influence of the human element, the use of quantitative measures is encouraged. Quantification is believed to be value-free and is used to supply unimpeded access to reality (Ellul, 1964). This claim is also sustained by the dualistic notion that things are either one way or the other (i.e., right or wrong, real or unreal, true or false) with no shades of gray. Stated simply, by becoming increasingly formalized, quantitative methods are assumed to be divorced from interpretation. Truth and objective reality are one.

Derived from rationalism, then, the cornerstone of the biomedical model is the materialization of life. Specifically, humans are approached as if they are simply physiological organisms. But this vision does not make much sense unless credence is given to several proposals. Dualism, empiricism, mechanical causality, the equilibrium thesis, and the neutrality of technique constitute the philosophical underside of biomedicine, and these philosophical themes are manifested in the five doctrines of the biomedical model.

THE DOCTRINES OF THE BIOMEDICAL MODEL

Freund and McGuire (1991) have argued that the ways in which the body is understood are socially constructed. There are cultural ideals *of* the body. No less important, however, are the philosophical developments *about* the body that are historically and culturally based. Emphasized in traditional Chinese medicine, for example, is the *chi* in the body whose balance and manipulation bring about health. This model is essentially non-material. In light of the previous discussion concerning historical philosophical development, there should be no surprise that in the West, by contrast, the body is understood to be essentially material, and the scientific approach to medicine is overwhelmingly objective and rational. Indeed, the Western biomedical model is predicated on five related doctrines.

The first to arise was *the doctrine of mind-body dualism*. This Cartesian formulation may have been useful as a starting point for biomedical science, but it is increasingly difficult to affirm in the modern practice of medicine. This doctrine is a barrier to understanding the psychosocial component of medicine, including the placebo effect, the connection between stress and illness, the importance of support groups, and the more general relationship between social support and health. Although the doctrine is no longer strictly adhered to, psychosomatic phenomena (i.e., the interaction between the mind and body) is still often considered to be peripheral to scientific medicine. In some contexts, this schism is actually an embarrassment, and many members of the medical science community seem ready for its reformulation. Patient-centered interviewing, for example, is becoming a common item in medical school curricula. This style of interviewing attends explicitly to psychosocial consequences and the illness experience of the patient, alongside a review of systems, history of current illness, and family health history.

The second doctrine is that the body is a system of functionally interdependent parts. Usually, this thesis is referred to as *the mechanical analogy,* whereby the body is treated as though it operates like a machine. Furthermore, the doctor is like a mechanic. The study of specific disease mechanisms makes up a considerable block of the usual medical school curriculum. Cassell (1991) has observed that the diagnosis of disease is normally based on the belief that each bodily function reflects a particular structure (e.g., kidney function/the biochemistry and anatomy of the kidney). So when disease is noticed, the structure of an organ is the first place to look for a cause, microscopic or otherwise. The search for tumors is predicated on this framework. The mechanical analogy is also invoked when the cardiovascular system is described as a hydraulic system and the heart as a muscle pump. Thinking that a physician can repair one part of the body removed from others, however, is quite a simplistic view.

Third is *the doctrine of physical reductionism.* Simply put, disease is viewed to be isomorphic with the malfunction of physiology. This focus on materialism excludes all non-material dimensions (social, psychological, and behavioral) in the search for causes, and therefore obscures the social conditions or physical environments that contribute to pathology or promote healing. Similar to body-mind dualism, context is denied. The answers are in the body alone. Reductionism is seen in the tendency to look for answers at progressively more *basic* levels, finally attempting to locate causes largely in the genes. The fourth doctrine is that the body is the appropriate focus of *regimen and control.* This principle is a logical corollary of physical reductionism. If disease exists in the body, then the body would be the logical locus of treatment. Because of the emphasis that is placed on physiology, a patient has the responsibility to follow the doctor's orders. After all, the physician is assumed to be an expert in this area. This doctrine is under great strain due to medical consumerism. In patient-centered interviewing courses, student doctors are encouraged to "negotiate" a treatment plan with the patient, an approach that would violate this doctrine, if employed broadly in future clinical practice.

And finally, or fifth, *the doctrine of specific etiology* relates to the idea that each disease has only one cause. This rendition of causality was strongly reinforced by germ theory and the invention of vaccines to attack the microbial origins of disease. The search for "magic bullet" cures which motivates most medical research is promoted by this doctrine.

This discussion of the biomedical model has remained at the theoretical level. Perhaps a better way to understand how philosophy has shaped medical practice is to examine briefly the rise of scientific medicine. Accordingly, the actual impact of certain concepts can be appreciated.

THE FLOWERING OF SCIENTIFIC MEDICINE

Scientific medicine developed as a result of adopting and applying science to medical concerns. In short, science came first. Biophysical science found its major applications in medicine, much as physics found its primary application in engineering.

The idea of scientific medicine can be traced back to the twelfth century B.C. to a Greek physician, Asclepias, whose followers believed that the chief duty of the physician was to treat disease and correct imperfections (Dubos, 1959). Disease theory, however, developed only recently in France in the early decades of the nineteenth century (Cassell,

1991). The classification of diseases was a conscious effort to introduce science into medicine. Having a universal classificatory scheme was viewed as essential for securing common understanding among doctors. A natural history approach, similar to classifying flora and fauna, was adopted. The attempt to describe diseases followed. Once diseases, which were viewed otologically as "things," were defined and consensus was gained on these definitions, the search for their causes, their etiology, could proceed apace. Structure and function were at the basis of the search for causes, and the mechanical analogy provided a unifying model of the causal chains. On the basis of a disease's classification, a physician could make diagnoses with regard to a generally accepted etiology. Indeed, a physician could prescribe a therapeutic treatment, or regimen, that would control and cure the disease. Disease classification, etiology, and treatment were disseminated throughout the medical profession, thereby supplying the basis for a consensus that eventually came to be equated with fact and truth.

The decades between 1800 and 1830 mark the shift away from philosophically based classical medicine to scientifically based clinical medicine. Perhaps better than any other event, the invention of the first crude stethoscope by Laennac in 1816 symbolizes the shift in perspective. Before, doctors observed patients but now they *examined* them (Starr, 1982). Furthermore, in Paris, the doctors began keeping statistics on the effectiveness of therapeutic techniques.

As scientific medicine developed into the mid-1800s, doctors became more detached and ignored the experience of patients, and instead paid attention to physiological markers. Ophthalmoscopes and laryngoscopes were added to stethoscopes to strengthen the physician's sensory powers in clinical examinations. A focus on the person was being supplanted by a focus on the body. When the microscope, X-ray, and chemical and bacteriological tests appeared, along with machines to measure physiological functioning, the transition was complete. The patient's subjective judgement was no longer needed. So-called objective evidence was viewed as much more accurate and reliable. The answers to disease were to be found in the body, not in the mind or the environment. The Cartesian doctrine of body-mind dualism, and the related theme of physical reductionism, had promoted the shift from person to body that flourished in the emerging science of medicine. In the background there were always great clinicians, such as William Osler, who never ignored the personhood of the patient. Increasingly, however, this more holistic emphasis gave way to scientific medicine's narrower focus on the body.

By the early 1900s, standardized rates and actuarial tables for comparing a patient to populations had been introduced to help physicians make objective judgments, based on the idea of normality. Eye charts, weight-height tables, and IQ tests are examples of the inventions of this period. In each case, normalcy is associated with objective criteria that are devoid of the uncertainty associated with subjectivity. Normal and abnormal, those dichotomous (or dualistic) concepts, came to reign supreme in clinical medicine and guide both diagnostic and treatment decisions.

In the 1880s, the organisms responsible for epidemic killers like tuberculosis, cholera, typhoid fever, and diphtheria were isolated. Microbiology allowed physicians to establish the links between disease and cause, between diagnosis and treatment, in a powerful way. So completely were these connections imprinted on the popular mind that germ theory, and the specific perspective on etiology of the biomedical model, came to dominate scientific medicine and raise hopes that disease would soon be eradicated from the earth, or at least from the civilized world. By the 1890s, medicine was actually making a difference in persons' health, although these improvements resulted mostly from prevention and other advancements in public health (Starr, 1982). The microscope became the symbolic logo of medical research, just as the stethoscope had become for clinical medicine (Reisner, 1978).

Antiseptic surgery was invented by Joseph Lister in 1867. This method was not perfected and applied broadly until the last decades of the century when virtuoso surgeons such as Charles and William Mayo gained celebrity status, raising hopes, again, for miraculous outcomes from common killers such as appendicitis and gall bladder disease.

When Abraham Flexner of the Carnegie Foundation visited medical schools and wrote his famous *Bulletin Number Four* in 1910, scientific medicine became the primary mode of investigating and treating disease. Flexner argued that all medical schools should be closed except those that trained the scientist-physician. Johns Hopkins and Harvard, rooted in basic science and hospital medicine, were to be the models. This reorganization of medical education had implications beyond the training of physicians. The entire edifice of professional medicine took shape. These changes were consistent with the rise of positivism and the belief in its ability to procure objectively valid knowledge. The result has been the cultural legitimation and dominance of scientific medicine, whose aim was to conquer disease. Doctors trained after 1920, on the whole, have a hard time distinguishing between science and medicine. To be sure, medicine's total embrace of science has had profound effects. Nonetheless, by the end of the twentieth century, the orthodox biomedical model would be challenged by the clinical demands posed by the growth of the older population in the United States.

PARADIGM STRAIN AND MEDICAL POLITICS

Pressures on the biomedical model and scientific medicine have come from several quarters, primarily during the second half of the twentieth century. Psychology, and particularly psychiatry, have understood the mind-body connection for the entire twentieth century and their influence in medicine has been gradual but continuous. An association for psychosomatic medicine became visible in the 1950s, made up of physicians who openly challenged the mind-body dualism doctrine of the biomedical model, and it foreshadowed developments two decades later.

As the nation's level of education increased, the general population was less impressed than before by the "miracles" of science. The failures of science were also evident. "Better things for better living through chemistry" became a hollow slogan to those who were aware of the ways in which chemicals were poisoning the environment. Science is not the beneficent force that it once had seemed. The environmental movement contributed to eroding the status that science once held.

The loss of wonder at the progress of science seems to have come in the 1960s and early 1970s when authority of all kinds was being challenged by a baby boom come of age. Medical authority did not escape its challenge. Physicians seemed less like gods and their sovereign profession came increasingly under fire as a fortification for greed. The escalating cost of medicine, and dwindling access to it, served to underscore a public sense of betrayal by both science and professional medicine. Scientific medicine, to skeptics, looked like the monopolization of professional knowledge, an excuse for keeping prices high and avoiding competition.

The environmental movement and the challenge to institutional authority were corrosive factors on the unquestioned power and orthodoxy of scientific medicine. In the meantime, the values that infused the consumer protection movement were reshaping the doctor-patient relationship. The detachment that physicians had gained in the scientific pursuit of disease seemed to have eroded the personal relationship that, at least in folklore, bonded the doctor to the patient. Dependence on objective laboratory tests, rather than subjectively recounting the symptoms and life circumstances by patients, made the doctor and patient less accessible to one another as persons. Scientific detachment was no longer offset by unquestioning trust in the scientist-physician by their patients. Corporate medicine may have created the circumstances, and the consumer protection movement the values, but the fact remains that the prevailing approach to medicine is commercial, with medical care viewed as a commodity, provided by physicians, with patients as the consumers. The values and attitudes that subtend commercial relationships are pragmatic and self-interested, and not idealistic. This shift erodes further the unquestioned authority of the physician.

In the midst of these cultural changes in the United States, there was a population change occurring that would form the greatest challenge of all to the Western biomedical model–the population of the nation was aging.

Population aging has such a strong effect on medicine because health issues change during the life course. Epidemiologist Maurice Mittelmark (1993) made this point clearly when he asserted that "accident and injury are prominent concerns in childhood, adolescence and early adulthood, developing chronic diseases are a central feature of middle adulthood, morbidity and mortality from chronic diseases characterize the period around retirement, and deterioration in functioning, disability and dependency are concerns mainly of old and very old age" (p. 3).

The aging of the population shifts the emphasis from acute disease, accidents, and injuries to chronic disease, and deterioration in functioning. Chronic diseases such as heart disease, Alzheimer's, and diabetes, and chronic conditions such as hypertension, osteoporosis, and osteoarthritis can be managed, but they cannot be cured. Furthermore, with advancing old age, chronic diseases and conditions tend to accumulate. The medical care of older adults, therefore, focuses on the *management* of chronic disease, and increasingly on rehabilitation, but rarely on *cure*. The original aim of scientific medicine to discover and conquer disease is thereby sidetracked.

Cracks from paradigm strain are now visible in the edifice of the Western biomedical model. It is possible to point to some of the features of an emerging paradigm: one that will be responsive to the health of the growing elderly population. In some circles, this new philosophy is referred to as post-quantum theory, while in others the term is postmodernism. At the core of either viewpoint, however, is the rejection of dualism.

THE EMERGING PARADIGM

The emerging paradigm represents a change toward a much greater emphasis on the "biopsychosocial" viewpoint that disease occurs because of interaction between persons and their environment (Foss & Rothenberg, 1987). If diseases are things, in the ontological sense, then they should have a discrete beginning and end. But disease categories are abstractions; they are human inventions; they have no independent existence. They are also static. On the other hand, the story of an illness, including the conditions that contributed to it (within and outside the body), is found in the life-world of the patient. Pathophysiology, in short, is dynamic. Therefore, most chronic diseases or conditions make more sense when viewed within a framework that elevates in importance values, commitments, desires, biography, and other interpretive considerations.

Cassel (1991) attributes much of the early theoretical work on the emerging paradigm to Rene Dubos, who began to write increasingly in the late 1950s and throughout the 1960s about the interdependence of organisms and their environments. In his book *The Mirage of Health* (1959), he argued that the claim that the tubercula bacillus, for example, is the *cause* of tuberculosis, in the absence of environmental factors, is naive in the extreme. Intestinal microbes are omnipresent in humans; their attack is triggered by changes in the internal (bodily) and external environments, which are themselves interdependent and evolving. In this way, the body was united inextricably to a wider web of nonphysiological considerations. Disease, accordingly, is not autonomous and something that simply attacks the body.

Imagine a case conference in a medical school. The case presented by a professor of internal medicine is about a man, age 78, who was found unconscious by a neighbor in his fifth-floor walk-up apartment in the inner city. When he reached the emergency room, a quick chest examination pointed to pneumonia as the presenting illness. The attending physician expected that the pneumonia was caused by the pneumococcus, a belief later confirmed. The patient was thus treated with penicillin. One of his knees was also swollen, which turned out to be the result of osteoarthritis. He responded well to the drug therapy; his fever came down; his lungs cleared and he was released to go home. This appeared to be an example of successful scientific medicine.

The case seemed uninteresting to the interns and residents. The diagnosis had been quick and straightforward, the treatment was appropriate, and the patient got well without complications. "But there is more," said the professor. "It is artificial to stop at the boundaries of the body. There is a story here, and none of you discovered it because you did not ask all of the right questions." The man's grief at the loss of his wife caused him to be depressed. He was socially isolated; no social support was available to him. He lived alone and kept to himself since his wife died. The depression caused a loss of appetite. The swollen knee made it very painful to descend and ascend the stairs, so he did not go out for groceries. Malnutrition resulted, which weakened his immune system and made him vulnerable to bacterial infections. Pneumonia resulted.

That is half of the story. In his "aloneness" and sorrow, he began drinking one night, became intoxicated, vomited, aspirated the vomitus into his lungs and developed a lung abscess or aspiration pneumonia, and he was brought back to the emergency room just two weeks after his release. The students again talked about diagnosis and treatment. The professor shook his head. "Don't you get it?" he said. "By limiting your view only to the disease state, you are missing the other factors in the story. His solitude, his bereavement, his living conditions, his bad knee, his nutrition, *and* the pneumococcus infection, antibiotics and respirator, are *all* part of the story. The search for the cause of an illness is limited by the classic disease theory. It does not account for all of the facts and until you understand this, you may be able to get a patient out of a hospital, but you cannot keep him out for very long." This hypothetical example, drawn largely from Cassel's examination of the nature of human suffering and the goals of medicine (1991), illustrates the paradigm strain.

This more encompassing strategy is justified by recent developments in philosophy. Metanarratives, as Lyotard (1984) uses the term, are scenarios that claim an absolute status, because they are believed to be sustained by Divine inspiration, natural law, or some other factor that is immune to situational contingencies. Biomedicine is replete with metanarratives; pathogens, the body, the disease state, and health are often treated as autonomous. These are simply realities that members of the medical team are trained to recognize.

The reason why metanarratives are rejected is quite simple. Due to recent shifts in understanding language use, objectivity cannot be separated clearly from subjectivity. Derrida's (1976) infamous phrase, "nothing exists outside of the text," captures this view of knowledge. Language does not merely point to objects, but mediates everything that is known. Language cannot be placed aside. Because there is no escape from interpretation, Descartes' dream is shattered (Bordo, 1987). This subversion of dualism has implications for medicine that are difficult to ignore. Take the body, for instance. Because interpretation is ubiquitous, discomfort, pain, or illness should not be associated exclusively with the presence of standard physiological markers. Within this framework, the body and mind are inextricably united; the person is not merely a physiological organism. In this regard, every bodily sign is psychosomatic, and not simply those that cannot be readily explained by biomedicine (Murphy & Longino, 1992).

In general, facts are not objective in the dualistic sense, but are thought to reside within a person's *Lebenswelt* or "life-world." This term indicates that facts are embroiled in the values, beliefs, and commitments. In terms of the *Lebenswelt,* a single empirical referent can have several meanings depending on how reality is constructed by a patient. What is considered to be significant is thus situationally prescribed.

Viewed from within the life-world, patients are persons who are connected to an environment that has meaning. Forgetting to tell the social side of an apparently objective causal sequence, accordingly, will obscure the human element that ties variables together. The residents and interns mentioned earlier failed to recognize that the strength of the relationship between factors depends on how persons view themselves, others, and the social context. What appeared to them to have a straightforward cause and solution was actually a much more complex problem.

In biomedicine, technical refinement is thought to lead to an improved knowledge base, which can be used to upgrade the intervention process. Improved technique, however, does not automatically make a researcher more aware of how reality is interpreted. For this reason, Habermas (1970) argues that the principle of "communicative competence" should guide research. Researchers should attempt to become value relevant. A physician, accordingly, should try to gain entree to a patient's worldview in order to clarify a diagnosis, rather than rely on more laboratory tests.

In sum, the biomedical model is under siege by many philosophers. With respect to identifying health and illness, interpretation must be recognized to pervade the practice of medicine. Because disease is implicated in a cultural dynamic that pervades the body and every other facet of life, physicians should attend to the experiential nature of a patient's problem. Patients also define their condition, in addition to physicians. Therefore, the issue is to create a situation where both viewpoints are given credence.

The Western biomedical model delegitimizes the power of persons to define themselves in the face of pressure from the medical establishment to provide "objective" definitions. Even though physicians are hardly objective, operating as they do according to the culture of science, they demand submission from patients. This position is no longer warranted, however, from a point of view that begins with the person and not the body. The view that medicine must be democratized is specifically important if a biopsychosocial view of medicine is ever inaugurated on a large scale.

PARADIGM SHIFT AND POLICY CHANGE

Democratizing medicine seems congenial to a culture that is said to espouse individualistic values. As Jean Gebser (1985) declares, "the center is everywhere." There would be no longer any places where absolutes, such as those fostered by biomedicine, could hide. Absolutes are merely modes of interpretation that have gained widespread acceptance. As noted by Roland Barthes (1986), objectivity is a special case of language use.

Many aspects of medical care would have to be rethought if dualism were honestly rejected (Foss & Rothenberg, 1987). Types of medicine competing with one another in a pluralistic environment was characteristic of America during the early and middle nineteenth century (Starr, 1982). Orthodox biomedicine only came to dominate the medical scene almost completely in the twentieth century. A postmodernist philosophy of medicine would undermine medical orthodoxy, encouraging once again input from various members of a community without fear that the practice of medicine would be ruined.

Furthermore, health care is mostly shaped by medical knowledge. When making a diagnosis, for example, a patient's suggestions are not given much credence. Intuition, simply put, is not thought to be scientific and is dismissed as invalid (Kestenbaum, 1982). Abandoning dualism, however, fosters a more encompassing approach to assessment. A diverse body of knowledge can be introduced, thereby allowing a host of options to be tested before a final recommendation is made. For there is no reason *a priori,* related to value-freedom or tradition, for limiting input to biomedicine. The interdisciplinary nature of geriatric assessment seems to the most orthodox to be a step in the direction of democratizing medicine. From the stand staked out by postmodern theory, however, this attempt to be pluralistic would be only a small step in the direction of democratization.

On topics less directly related to the power of the medical profession, a postmodern philosophy of medicine seems more relevant. The mind, biography, surrounding environment, and culture, for instance, are a few considerations that become very significant in a non-Cartesian world. Given the unity of subjectivity and objectivity, the locus of intervention should extend beyond the confines of physical nature.

Physicians are blamed regularly for overmedicating patients. But considering the prevailing dualistic image of the body, this method of treatment makes sense. Due to the obsession with disease, non-medical options are assumed to be fraudulent. Treatment can be redefined, however, so that medicine can become more culturally sensitive. Chiropractic and folk medicine, for example, would no doubt begin to play a larger role in treatment, as they did before the hegemony of orthodox medicine in the United States.

Biomedicine has fostered some practices that have become problematic. The body became an object that could be known accurately only by technical, medical experts. In the end, the human character of illness was eclipsed, while medical practice was shrouded by authority and removed from public view.

The praxis of an anti-dualistic philosophy of medicine, therefore, would focus on empowerment through a change in culture and self. This philosophical stance would argue that people must begin to believe that their body is not an object that operates solely according to the laws of nature, and that social and cultural correctives can be undertaken that promote health. In other words, health care should no longer be viewed as within the sole purview of physicians and drug companies. Furthermore, persons would be urged to believe that they have a right to the knowledge that has been reserved for medical experts alone. In this way, real prevention programs could be inaugurated. In general, persons would be given the latitude to participate fully in every facet of their treatment, from defining health to making a diagnosis.

CONCLUSION

Tempering the biomedical model, excepting it in certain circumstances, is not a paradigm shift. Neither is the observation that the sovereignty of professional medicine is waning sufficient. These are examples of paradigm *strain,* cracks in the walls of the Western biomedical edifice, and the vast industry that has grown up around it.

A true shift from a dualistic to an anti-dualistic paradigm would require that something quite different would have to be erected in its place. Such dramatic alterations may someday occur, inch by inch if not suddenly. Postmodern philosophy would promote these changes.

R. D. Laing (1973) once claimed that psychiatric patients would probably be helped more by an epistemologist than a psychiatrist. There is a sense in which epistemology and practice cannot be separated. One implies the other. The movement that has been witnessed during the past twenty years and has challenged the biomedical model and broadened the scope of medicine is supported by certain epistemological principles that are difficult to ignore. And if this epistemological side of medicine is given serious consideration, a new approach to delivering medical care may be on the horizon. This conclusion may sound strange to those who believe that medicine is an especially practical discipline. Nonetheless, a change in philosophical worldview is essential to a socially responsive approach to medicine.

REFERENCES

Barthes, R. (1986). *The rustle of language.* New York: Hill and Wang.

Bordo, S.R. (1987). *The flight to objectivity.* Albany: SUNY Press.

Carlson, R.J. (1975). *The end of medicine.* New York: John Wiley and Sons.

Cassel, E.J. (1991). *The nature of suffering and the goals of medicine.* New York: Oxford University Press.

Derrida, J. (1976). *Of grammatology.* Baltimore: Johns Hopkins University Press.

Dubos, R. (1959). *Mirage of health: Utopias, progress, and biological change.* Garden City: Doubleday & Company, Inc.

Ellul, J. (1964). *The technological society.* New York: Random House.

Foss, L. & Rothenberg, K. (1987). *The second medical revolution.* Boston: Shambhala.

Foucault, M. (1989). *The archaeology of knowledge.* London: Routledge.

Gebser, J. (1985). *The ever-present origin.* Athens: Ohio University Press.

Habermas, J. (1970). Towards a theory of communicative competence. In H.P. Dreitzel (Ed.), *Recent sociology* (2nd ed.) (pp. 115-148). New York: Macmillan.

Kestenbaum, V. (1982). Introduction: The experience of illness. In V. Kestenbaum (Ed.), *The humanity of the ill* (pp. 13-20). Knoxville: The University of Tennessee Press.

Laing, R.D. (1973). The mystification of experience. In P. Brown (Ed.), *Radical psychology* (pp. 109-127). New York: Harper and Row.

Lyotard, J.F. (1984). *The postmodern condition: A report on knowledge.* Minneapolis: University of Minnesota Press.

Mittelmark, M.B. (1993). The epidemiology of aging. In W.L. Hazzard, E.L. Birman, J.P. Blass, W.H. Ettinger, & J.B. Halter (Eds.), *Principles of geriatric medicine and gerontology.* New York: McGraw-Hill, Inc. In press.

Murphy, J.W. & Longino, C.F., Jr. (1992). What is the justification for a qualitative approach to ageing studies? *Ageing and society, 12,* 143-156.

Norell, S. (1984). Models of causation in epidemiology. In L. Nordenfelt & B.I.B. Lindahl (Eds.), *Health, disease, and causal explanation in medicine.* Dordrecht: Dusseldorf.

Reisner, S.J. (1978). *Medicine and the reign of technology.* London: Cambridge University Press.

Schwartz, M.A. & Wiggins, O.P. (1988). Scientific and humanistic medicine: A theory of clinical methods. In K.L. White (Ed.), *The task of medicine.* Menlo Park: The Henry J. Kaiser Family Foundation.

Starr, P. (1982). *The social transformation of American medicine: The rise of a sovereign profession and the making of a vast industry.* New York: Basic Books.

Strasser, H. & Randall, S.C. (1981). *An introduction to theories of social change.* London: Routledge and Kegan Paul.

Weber, M. (1978). *Economy and society: Vol I.* Berkeley: University of California Press.

Weber, M. (1958). *The Protestant ethic and the spirit of capitalism.* New York: Scribners.

Index

Aristotle
 reason, 10
artificial intelligence
 description of, 12

Babbage, Charles
 reason, 12
Barthes, Roland
 objectivity, 114
behaviorism
 epistemology of, 37-38
biomedical model
 and anti-dualism, 114; and the
  biopsychosocial viewpoint,
  110-112; chronic disease,
  102; critique of, 106-109;
  history of, 102-105;
  implementation of, 106-109;
  key characteristics of, 54,
  103-104; and the life-world,
  112-113; mechanical
  analogy, 105; mind-body
  dualism, 105; physiological
  reductionism, 106; and
  reason, 7; regimen and
  control; specific etiology,
  106
biopsychosocial viewpoint
 description of, 110-112
Boole, George
 reason, 12
bounded rationality
 description of, 40

Cassell, Eric J.

mind-body dualism, 105; critique
 of the biomedical model,
 111,112
Chopra, Deepak, 55
cognitive behaviorist theory
 critique of, 34-35
Colby, Kenneth
 computerized interviews, 25
communicative competence
 description of, 16,113
community-based research
 and community planning, 59; and
  data gathering, 62; and
  dualism, 61; key elements
  of, 58; and the life-world,
  61; limitations of, 62-63; a
  new approach to medicine,
  59; new model of the
  universe, 60; and
  objectivity, 61;
  questionnaire design, 61;
  and reductionism, 61-62
computer technology
 and client interviews, 25; context of
  utilization, 26-29; and
  decision-making, 41;
  information processing,
  40-41; information recording,
  21-22; and inventory testing,
  20-21; the language of
  computers, 20; management
  information system, 22-24;
  recommendations for the
  proper use of, 26-29; and
  research design, 25; and
  treatment plans, 21; word
  processing, 21
culture of science, 2-3

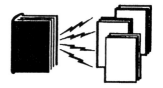

Haworth
DOCUMENT DELIVERY
SERVICE

This valuable service provides a single-article order form for any article from a Haworth journal.

- *Time Saving:* No running around from library to library to find a specific article.
- *Cost Effective:* All costs are kept down to a minimum.
- *Fast Delivery:* Choose from several options, including same-day FAX.
- *No Copyright Hassles:* You will be supplied by the original publisher.
- *Easy Payment:* Choose from several easy payment methods.

Open Accounts Welcome for . . .
- Library Interlibrary Loan Departments
- Library Network/Consortia Wishing to Provide Single-Article Services
- Indexing/Abstracting Services with Single Article Provision Services
- Document Provision Brokers and Freelance Information Service Providers

MAIL or *FAX* THIS ENTIRE ORDER FORM TO:

Haworth Document Delivery Service
The Haworth Press, Inc.
10 Alice Street
Binghamton, NY 13904-1580

or **FAX:** 1-800-895-0582
or **CALL:** 1-800-342-9678
9am-5pm EST

PLEASE SEND ME PHOTOCOPIES OF THE FOLLOWING SINGLE ARTICLES:
1) Journal Title: _____
   Vol/Issue/Year: _____ Starting & Ending Pages: _____
   Article Title: _____

2) Journal Title: _____
   Vol/Issue/Year: _____ Starting & Ending Pages: _____
   Article Title: _____

3) Journal Title: _____
   Vol/Issue/Year: _____ Starting & Ending Pages: _____
   Article Title: _____

4) Journal Title: _____
   Vol/Issue/Year: _____ Starting & Ending Pages: _____
   Article Title: _____

(See other side for Costs and Payment Information)

COSTS: Please figure your cost to order quality copies of an article.

1. Set-up charge per article: $8.00
   ($8.00 × number of separate articles) _____

2. Photocopying charge for each article:
   1-10 pages: $1.00 _____

   11-19 pages: $3.00 _____

   20-29 pages: $5.00 _____

   30+ pages: $2.00/10 pages _____

3. Flexicover (optional): $2.00/article _____

4. Postage & Handling: US: $1.00 for the first article/
   $.50 each additional article _____

   Federal Express: $25.00 _____

   Outside US: $2.00 for first article/
   $.50 each additional article_____

5. Same-day FAX service: $.35 per page _____

GRAND TOTAL: _____

METHOD OF PAYMENT: (please check one)

❑ Check enclosed   ❑ Please ship and bill. PO # _____
(sorry we can ship and bill to bookstores only! All others must pre-pay)

❑ Charge to my credit card: ❑ Visa; ❑ MasterCard; ❑ Discover;
❑ American Express;

Account Number:_____ Expiration date:_____

Signature: **✗**_____

Name: _____ Institution: _____

Address: _____

_____

City: _____ State:_____ Zip:_____

Phone Number: _____ FAX Number: _____

MAIL or *FAX* THIS ENTIRE ORDER FORM TO:

Haworth Document Delivery Service	**or FAX:** 1-800-895-0582
The Haworth Press, Inc.	**or CALL:** 1-800-342-9678
10 Alice Street	9am-5pm EST)
Binghamton, NY 13904-1580	